MEDITATION FOR MEDICS: STOPPING THE NOISE

A SIMPLE GUIDE TO UNSHAKEABLE MINDFULNESS BY A BUSY ER DOCTOR

DR ANDREW DEAN

Dean, Dr Andrew

Meditation for Medics: Stopping the Noise - A Simple Guide to Unshakeable Mindfulness by a Busy ER Doctor

ISBN: 978-1-7637882-7-5

CONTENTS

FROM THE AUTHOR

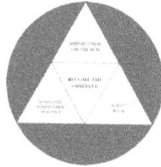

This book has been written for clinicians. Firstly, for my ED/ER doctor colleagues, but also for medical students, nurses, and other healthcare workers.

As doctors and nurses, especially in critical care environments – or in my case the Emergency Department - we are constantly surrounded by *noise* - environmental noise (outside us), internal noise (our own busy thoughts that keep us preoccupied), and emotional noise in the form of our internal reactions to the environment.

This *noise* does not of itself create stress; rather, it's our reaction to these *triggers* that creates such potential for negative stress and anxiety.

Stress and anxiety detract from our quality of life. They stop us finding a sense of peace and experiencing joy in each moment. Burn-out and psychological trauma may result. They also make it harder to do our job well.

This book is about learning the art of *unshakeable mindfulness*, the ability to stop the mental noise when stress and anxiety start to take hold of us.

Unshakeable mindfulness has been a core element of my life and work delivery as an ER doctor for almost 40 years. It is what I practice daily in emergency room environments and has become an integral part of what I teach to junior doctors and medical students.

Emergency medicine and clinical reasoning are by nature and necessity always based on 'hard science', as the ER is no place for alternative medicine. However, in every respect good clinical practice is *augmented* by mindfulness.

I have practised these simple and accessible techniques for many years, and I share them in the hope that they will enable you also to find calmness, and a deeper sense of fulfilment not only in clinical work, but also externally in your "other" life.

Dr Andrew Dean
Emergency Physician
MB BS, FACEM, Grad Cert Clinical Simulation
October 2025

A DAY IN THE ER...

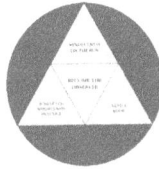

It was 2.00pm on a Wednesday and the ER was already busy. The retrieval call came in on the red phone. The paramedics needed a doctor and nurse to go to help rescue a hiker. She had slipped off the path on a sloping rock face and had injured her ankle and hit her head. She had been unconscious briefly, but had regained consciousness and remained alert. We didn't yet know about potential chest, spinal or pelvic injuries.

The paramedics had identified a large laceration on her head. We collected our medications for pain relief, also the anaesthetic intubation drugs, and a range of other airway equipment, C collars, splints, and wound dressings. What was not known was whether we would need to intubate and ventilate her in preparation for the 250 km (160 mile) helicopter flight back to a large city trauma hospital.

A retrieval nurse and I walked out from the ER, and loaded our gear and ourselves into the waiting ambulance. There were "lights and sirens" through the town, then once we reached the open road, the ambulance travelled at around 120 kmh (75mph).

The mountain range where she fell was nearly 150 km (90 miles) from our hospital, with the last part on dirt roads leading into a National Park.

Ambulances are not known for comfort - they are heavy vehicles with matching suspension. We were holding on around each corner as the medical monitoring equipment strained against its straps. We had some early information from the on-site paramedics that our patient had a possible compound skull fracture, as well as the laceration, so I started to plan the various treatment options. There were a range of possible options for her injuries, each with emergency interventions.

We would be carrying our gear up the rock face, and I already knew the steepness of that track. It was late afternoon when we arrived, heading into darkness.

The retrieval helicopter was airborne already, so I had to plan time-effective interventions to stabilise the patient pre-flight. The doctor at a retrieval is expected to anticipate and treat any emergency that arises at the scene.

I was feeling anxious, not knowing if, given the circumstances and rough terrain, I would be able to successfully deliver any treatment that the patient required.

A retrieval mission is a very public space, with patients, family members, paramedics and other emergency responders watching the doctor perform. I withdrew from the conversation between the paramedics and our ER nurse. I needed quiet time, to think it through, to plan the initial primary survey at the mountain, and the "Plan B" options for any other life-saving treatments that she might need.

The sun was going down as we drove, and I knew we would probably not arrive until near sunset. Climbing boulders in darkness with medical gear has its own risks. Still in our hospital scrubs, we were not dressed for outdoor trekking or climbing over rocks, and the retrieval pack itself was bulky to carry.

When we got to the base of the mountain, there was a 15-minute hike across sandy desert, and then a steep scramble upwards across craggy trees and boulders to where we ascended onto the rock-face itself. The helicopter was going to meet us there. Already, the first responders were present, working to comfort the injured hiker and provide first aid.

The scramble up the rocks was harder than we anticipated, especially in our hospital shoes. Even with the paramedics' help, the weight of the retrieval backpack was slowing us down. Across the fields we glimpsed an orange sunset developing. We knew we must get past the steep section before complete darkness descended. We were told that the helicopter had an ETA of 30 minutes. It would all come down to assessing the patient's stability. Airway establishment, ventilation for a head injury, ongoing sedation for the helicopter trip, IV fluids, antibiotics, and analgesia... which options would she need?

A calm mind in this situation is everything. Procedural skills and resuscitation capability are important. I am used to stabilising patients in a calm, well-lit environment without trees and a steep rock-face. This situation requires a different type of stillness and planning. The real help comes from reaching a place of mental clarity, or what I call an unshakeable mindfulness, that allows me to completely focus only on the task at hand.

The patient was already on an extrication sled, ready for lifting across the uneven rock to a winch point. I put in an IV cannula, *and we gave some morphine. The woman seemed alert, and the large laceration on her head had been covered with a temporary bandage dressing. I had a look, because the initial report had been of exposed brain tissue beneath the laceration. Fortunately, as I opened the bandage it was evident that the wound only went down to the level of the scalp muscle. Her ankle was probably fractured, but it too had first-aid splinting in place, and on this mountainside, there was nothing else I could really add.*

The helicopter arrived and the pilot was hovering above us, carefully training two overlapping spotlights onto the cliff face, to help judge the distance from the rock, as she held the chopper directly above us. The winch operator had extended the lifting frame and was in constant radio contact with the paramedics next to our patient. We were all in complete darkness now, except for various spotlights, navigation lights and ground-lights at set points to help orientate the pilot. I had one role, focussing on the safety of the hiker, as around me the winching operation began, in a well-rehearsed sequence. Watching a retrieval flight-crew in action is impressive.

Down came a flight paramedic on the cable, and he brought with him the lifting harness and extrication sled. With spinal precautions we lifted her across and the flight paramedic checked the harness straps, while I tried to explain to the patient what was going on. The rotor noise made that virtually impossible. The pilot was working hard to keep the light beams on top of each other so that the helicopter remained above us at a constant height of around 20 metres. Eventually, the winch began, and the hiker ascended slowly to the relative safety of the interior of the 'chopper'.

And then it was done. The helicopter curled around in a wide arc, climbing slowly, navigation lights flashing red and green as it started the long trip back to a trauma hospital.

The packing up and climbing down the mountain began. Strangely anti-climactic, but a good outcome for our patient...

"UNSHAKEABLE MINDFULNESS" – WHAT IS IT?

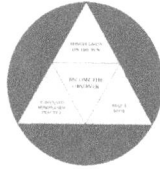

The mindset comes from being quiet. Taking control of the situation – perhaps a resuscitation in the ER in my world, or a different scene in your own life. Regardless of the situation – chaos and stress are universal, and our ability to create positive outcomes depends on how well we can navigate our way to the other side. It's about demanding that our mind follows instruction. It's about strength of mind and the ability to make the right decisions at the right time.

This requires unshakeable mindfulness.

Yet the power of mindfulness is also about nurture, of every person in the conversation. Seeing ourselves as responsible for those around us. Seeing ourselves as leaders.

So how do we reach this operating space?

We need to reduce the "noise" that our minds are so clever at generating. This book is about stopping that noise. The mental and emotional noise that pulls us out of our centre of stillness.

Unshakeable mindfulness is not some vague, new age concept. It's a skill. It needs practice every day.

To do this we need a strategy and action plan that can deliver on that. My strategy for achieving unshakeable mindfulness is through meditation. Effective and deliberate meditation reins in our mind and takes back control, in a gentle way, but also in a very determined way. As if our life depends on it.

Dr Jon Kabat-Zinn, a US physician and mindfulness pioneer, speaks also in these terms. He suggests that we "approach mindfulness and meditation as if our very life depends on it". He's right.

CONTENT OVERVIEW

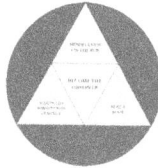

1. The Reasons

To change, to put in work, we need a *reason*. In emergency medicine, we learn quickly that achieving coordinated and effective action in a clinical care team, demands that we must first start with ourselves. Scene control in any resuscitation is crucial. The team members are affected by us as leaders; it is the crucial element that keeps the team cohesive, and it is proven to create a safer outcome for the sick or injured patient. This is the reason that good ER teams also need to think about unshakeable mindfulness as a deliberate approach. This applies to your life too. We will explore concepts of resilience and how important it is to see ourselves as *leaders in our own lives*, directing the traffic, managing the noise, and getting the outcomes we want.

2. Noise

Understanding noise is the first stage of changing our instinctive or 'default' reactions; we can't easily change external noise, but we can efficiently learn how to bring a rapid calmness to our internal and emotional noise. This the basis for mindfulness, especially in a busy clinical environment.

3. Silence

The idea that we can change our reaction patterns is a new idea to many people. Often, we assume that our emotions and our internal "chatter" are outside of our control, and we bounce along in the same state for most of our lives. It's exhausting. If we make the decision to do so, we can learn to efficiently reduce our inner *noise*.

4. Skills Development

In emergency medicine the skills that save a life need to be learned and regularly practiced to become instinctive. As with other skills in life, we learn by watching an expert, by attending courses or studying, and then by practising each day. *Unshakeable mindfulness* is simply another type of skill that is learned with practice, very similar to working in the ER. However, changing the patterns in our brain requires work and commitment. We look at the specifics of pushing past our "default reaction patterns", and rapidly reaching a *stillness space*.

5. Checklists

Nothing happens without preparation. There are several elements that create success with meditation and mindfulness. There are the *cognitive* aspects–study and reading. Then there's the scheduled *daily practice*. If we don't practice, we don't improve. As mindfulness students, we need to become *observers*, not just of ourselves and how we are thinking and reacting to situations, but of the situation around us. We ask ourselves, "What is my best response here?" In the stressful environment of our retrieval mission, a clear focus and situational awareness can literally be the difference between life and death. Not just for the patient, but for all of us beneath the "hovering helicopter" of our day. With mental calmness, both during meditation, and as we go about our daily lives, building the skill of self-observation supports us to take our skills to the next level, as we work towards *unshakeable mindfulness'* in every situation.

6. Going Next Level

If we are to achieve what we want from our lives, we need to get serious about our own growth. *Unshakeable mindfulness* is an important pathway to self-transformation. We will discuss the elements that make great *leaders*, and the overlap between great leadership and mindfulness. As we practice the techniques discussed in this book, a *larger* picture emerges. We will look at our *function* in the world, and the integration of *unshakeable mindfulness* into a life that serves others as well as ourselves. Mindfulness becomes the means, but it also gives the *meaning* for making the journey to become our best selves.

MY OWN STORY

BY DR ANDREW DEAN

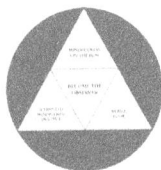

The idea of an emergency physician doctor writing a book about meditation, even while working in the ER and teaching medical students and young doctors, may seem unusual and strange. I am familiar with carrying the stress of my workplace home with me, and I have had to develop ways of thinking and practicing that enable me to become calm.

As with most things, necessity drives change.

When I contracted severe viral pneumonia several years ago, it was due to being burnt out by my long hours working in the ER, and also from combining clinical work with teaching duties.

In the midst of fever, sweating and chills, here I was, leaning heavily on a lecture theatre podium and giving a talk to medical students on multi-trauma assessment.

I was shocked that my insight and self-awareness had been so poor, particularly to push myself even further into the "red zone", by taking a commercial jet flight interstate, while already hypoxic from the developing pneumonia.

It was madness, to the point where a physician colleague admitted me through my own ER for a few days of enforced rest, oxygen, anti-viral medication and IV antibiotics. A real wake-up call.

The fact that I became ill to the point where I required admission to hospital for several days, caught me by surprise. I was completely out of balance, and yet still pushing myself to keep doing even more. As doctors we often do this, even when we have clear body signals to rest or seek our own health care.

I realised that I became burned out, not in one big moment, but slowly, quietly. Like many others in demanding roles, I kept showing up, kept pretending everything was fine... until it wasn't. Until my body started to fail me. Until I could no longer ignore the exhaustion and physical issues.

As doctors, we are trained to care for others. But I had to learn, the hard way, how to genuinely care for myself. Meditation became one of the most important tools in that healing process.

I'm telling this story not because it's unique, but because it's common. Too common. And if sharing what I've learned can help even one person avoid the slow slide into burnout, or find a way back from it, then it's worth telling.

We can't always change the system we work in. But we can change how we care for ourselves within it. And that begins with awareness. With honesty. And with the courage to pause and say, "There's another way."

I've come to understand, deeply and personally, the transformative power of meditation and the unshakeable mindfulness that it creates. It's not just a practice I lean on when things get tough; it's become a cornerstone of how I live and work.

As an emergency doctor, I work in an environment where we navigate high stakes situations daily, through chaos and noise; where seconds matter; and the pressure is relentless. Unshakeable mindfulness gives me something rare in my world, it allows me to meet chaos with calm, so I can stop the noise and sharpen my focus. It slows my heart rate, steadies my breath, calms my nervous system, and helps me think clearly when everything around me is urgent and every decision has consequence.

But more than that it has shaped who I am outside of the trauma bay. It grounds me and helps me navigate life with more clarity.

Meditation has improved my sleep, lowered my stress levels, and helped regulate the emotional whiplash that often comes with high-pressure work. It's strengthened my resilience, softened my reactivity, and brought more patience into my conversations, both with patients and the people I love.

It's taught me how to pause, how to respond instead of react, and how to reconnect with a deeper part of myself that isn't overwhelmed by every challenge that comes my way.

Meditation hasn't made life perfect. But it's made me stronger, clearer, calmer, and more present, as a doctor, and as a human being.

And in a world that often feels like it's noisy and spinning too fast, that is its own kind of medicine.

Seeing colleagues going through similar experiences made me realise that we must teach each other. Share our own stories.

And so, I'm sharing my story because I know I'm not the only one who's ever felt like they were running on empty. My own experience, and thinking about this whole area, finally evolved into the decision to write this book.

This is a guide book, squarely aimed at clinicians. It has a structure, as you have seen from the chapter headings, and we'll make a journey together in the coming pages, to progressively assemble the key ideas.

The journey will not only be about ideas but changing our habits of thinking and reacting. Transforming ourselves away from stressful emotional patterns, towards a version of ourselves that is less reactive, calmer and therefore better able to care for patients, colleagues and family.

This structural change in how we think and react requires our determination to "hold the space". It's about developing a combination of strength and stillness inside ourselves as clinicians, and meditation is one of the techniques that helps us to take back the control.

As a writer, and a doctor, I have a metaphorical foot planted in the "stress camp", but the other foot is increasingly seen standing in the "meditation camp". I can't say that I have mastered it all – I am not sure we ever do. I have "off" moments, where I fall back into my old patterns, but I can see the map better these days, to guide me rapidly back onto the path.

THE MINDFULNESS TRIANGLE

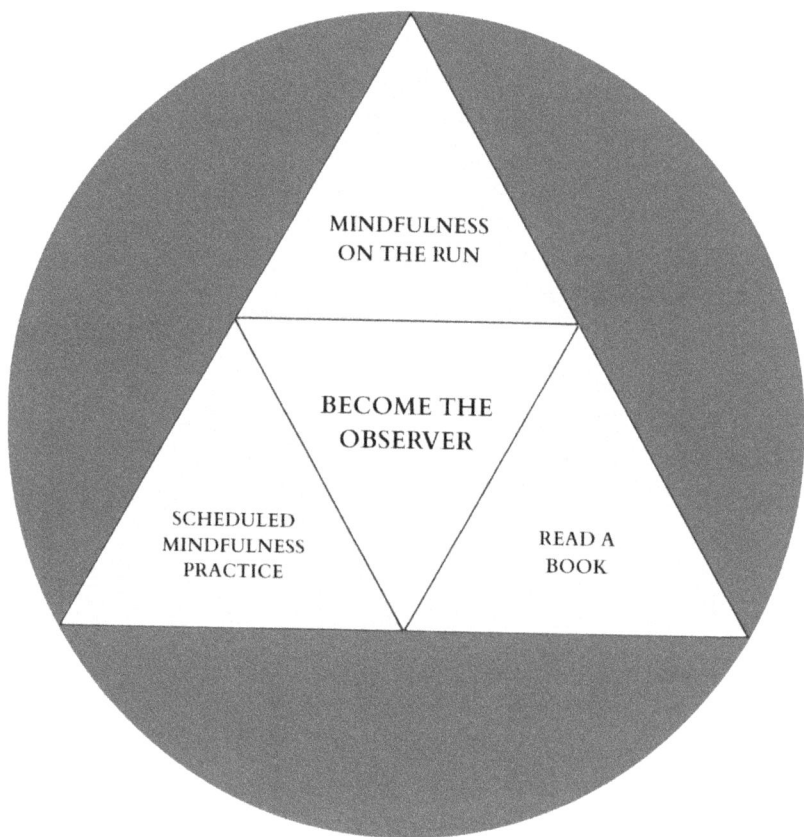

MINDFULNESS
ON THE RUN

BECOME THE
OBSERVER

SCHEDULED
MINDFULNESS
PRACTICE

READ A
BOOK

1

REASONS

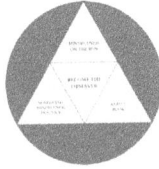

Another Friday morning in the ER and an elderly man comes in, with severe neck pain, holding his head at a strange angle. He is dependent on his wife for daily care due to advanced Parkinson's disease, and neck spasms are a common occurrence for him. It might have been a strain, but his wife was worried that he was more agitated than usual. So what was going on?

The nurses went through their assessment routines, making him as comfortable as they could. We inserted an IV and started analgesia. His pain and irritability were at extreme levels. I could feel my own stress building; I had never seen this before and the doses of morphine and fentanyl seemed way beyond what I would have expected.

But why? Pure musculoskeletal causes seemed less likely because of the sheer pain level. An unusual radiation of MI pain? ECG was normal. Perhaps a dissection in his aorta or his vertebral artery. Even meningitis was on the differential.

The process of thinking clearly about the differential diagnosis possibilities can be hard at the best of times, but amidst his screaming in pain I was feeling significant reactive anxiety myself. It clearly mattered that we get this right. Calm down and think.

The diagnostic thinking can be a lonely place for a doctor. With all the amazing support we have from the nurses, in the end it's on us, especially if the diagnosis is elusive.

Unshakeable mindfulness – that same theme returns. The reason why it mattered on this particular day was that, amidst the noise of this poor man with severe neck pain, I needed to find a very calm place to enable clear diagnostic thinking. It's like a map, and it helps us plan the next steps forward with investigations and treatment.

So that's the reason for the mindfulness training. We go to an opposite place. It matters. And even if my mind registers the natural stressful reaction to someone screaming in pain, I can still find a stillness.

The logic of how we established his diagnosis takes shape. Selecting the most useful blood tests, putting him on a sepsis pathway just in case, administering IV antibiotics early, with IV antiviral drugs to cover herpetic encephalitis. But first we needed to control the pain, and eventually we started to reach this point.

Results started to come back. His white cell count is twice the upper range of normal, and the CRP is a staggering 255 (the normal range here is under 3). There was an infection somewhere, and the thinking changed. Where? We targeted scans to the brain and neck. The brain CT scan was essentially normal with no bleed or tumour. But the neck scan suggests something unusual – a spreading abscess infection along the cervical spinal cord.

An MR scan followed, which revealed an epidural abscess lying in front of the spinal cord in his neck. The cord itself appeared inflamed and swollen on the scan. Discussions with neurosurgeons followed. Under advice, I attempted a spinal tap to sample the cerebrospinal fluid but didn't succeed due to severe arthritis in his lumbar vertebrae.

But at least we had our answer, an epidural abscess. More discussions, with the patient, his family, and with the neurosurgeon. Do we need to transfer him for surgery? In the end, he stayed in our hospital, managed with high-dose antibiotics, and followed through carefully by the neurosurgeon.

Unshakeable mindfulness kept my head clear, to allow optimal clinical reasoning in a very stressful situation. Reasoning which helped find a diagnosis that I had certainly never seen before...

Reasons for Making this Journey

To make any changes in our lives, we need a reason. So, what are our motivators for change? And what are the common reasons why people get into mindfulness and meditation?

Two reasons. One is **curiosity**, and the other is **pain.**

Some of us are in a position where "life is basically working." Perhaps we are open-minded to ideas of mindfulness, meditation, and spirituality. They seem interesting, so we decide to explore them. This is the "curiosity group."

The (likely) larger group of people who start to explore mindfulness make that decision in response to some kind of crisis in their lives: a relationship breakup, the loss of a job, or perhaps developing a major illness. The suffering and pain experienced from such events is exhausting and causes significant physical and emotional turmoil.

Many have had that direct experience of "life falling apart," and the subsequent struggles to get back on track. Alternatively, we may be closely involved supporting someone else as they experience such events.

In this latter group, it is the high level of pain and suffering that moves some of these people toward a realisation that *there must be a better way.*" It can often take extreme psychological pain before we question our assumptions or consider the possibility that our worldview and default patterns of reaction are contributing to our pain.

In the ER, we see frustration and anger often, especially now post-COVID. Health systems generally are chronically stressful places. It shows up in our patients, our hospital staff, and certainly in the ER nurses and doctors.

So, the reasons are certainly there, for us ER docs and nurses to learn about meditation. Well, *two* primary reasons actually.

Firstly, for *preventing burnout and mental health problems* in ourselves, that are brought on by the stress of our workplace. The work itself is stressful, but more importantly it is our reactions to that stress that create anxiety, anger and sadness if we do not approach situations through a "mindfulness" focus.

But the second reason is that if we can become *beacons of calm* amidst the stress, we will start to become "rescuers" for those around us, be they staff or patients. You will influence behaviour around you, anger levels will reduce, and in fact, you will progressively realise that you are hardly seeing any anger around you or even within you.

Then mindfulness becomes "wired in" and with further practice, becomes a part of our DNA – hence this term "*unshakeable mindfulness*".

Two good reasons for getting into mindfulness:
(1) we reduce *burnout*, and
(2) we become *beacons of calm*

So, in a way, the question now changes completely.

It becomes not so much, "Why should I do mindfulness?" but rather, "Why not?"

I think we will all eventually face the same question, but the timing is widely variable. Many of us just aren't yet ready to seriously make that decision for internal change.

But we all have to make our own way, in our own time.

I can only speak from my own experiences, which tells me that - with hospitals being so stressed out currently - we *absolutely* need leaders in mindfulness in the ER workplace and beyond, to help the staff stay afloat emotionally and psychologically.

The decision to change...

So here I am,
It's cold sunrise, and
Mist slides down the valleys
As I breathe slowly in,
And slowly out.
The old patterns just aren't working.
My stress is off the scale.
So don't laugh,
I'm trying something new.
Getting up early, out in the garden,
Shivering, and practicing "stillness" -
whatever that actually is -
There has to be a better way,
and I am going to find it.

Concepts of Resilience

Meditation enables resilience to stress...

- But what does that **mean**?
- Why do we **need** to become more resilient?

We may see resilience as being a type of toughening-up process, putting on a kind of mental armour that protects us against the insults and stress that "life out there" hurls at us.

You may be familiar with the old image of the resilient Western cowgirl or cowboy on their horse, tough as nails, enduring hardships and bad weather - and various venomous snakes as well.

This view of mental resilience involves seeing ourselves as being *separate* from other people around us, and may involve ideas like "I can handle it, it's just water off a duck's back," or "I'm tough, I don't need anyone else."

While this is perhaps a demonstration of admirable courage, it is certainly *not* mindfulness but merely an *illusion* of resilience.

In emergency medicine (and medicine in general), we sadly see this illusion of resilience playing out repeatedly, because the seemingly resilient doctors and nurses can be the ones who unexpectedly commit suicide or develop a substance addiction.

Something is genuinely wrong with the "tough resilience" model. The "tough resilience" always hides something, and that something is often a mental-health need that has not been addressed. And yet this version of "resilience" is still regarded by some as a goal worth aiming for.

Powerful Tools

Mindfulness and meditations are just tools for inner exploration and rearranging the way we think and experience life. Powerful tools.

As it happens, we don't just experience life, we can create life outside us by the way we think. This idea seems radical, but it is another good reason why mindfulness practice creates a "smoother" external life of interactions with others. Calmness on the inside, calmness on the outside. We probably all know individuals who demonstrate this, who inspire us. The opposite is true: chaos on the inside, chaos on the outside. We probably all know people who live like that as well.

So, when we are ready, the mindfulness path beckons.

We can create life outside us by the way we think.

From a young age, I accepted the commonly held view that life *just happens to us*. It all speaks of a lack of control, a kind of randomness about life events coming along, and just bumping into us, perhaps knocking us over.

This view of life is commonly agreed, but it makes us feel a bit powerless in the whole process. In the ER, we treat many young men who punch walls out of frustration, causing a fractured hand as a result. Go figure. But it just keeps on happening.

The idea that we cannot exert any predictive control over our experiences in life is crazy when you think about it.

Here's a simple example which we can probably all relate to. We can *certainly* exert *predictive control* over the oncoming day's experience in a negative way—when we start our day feeling really upset or angry, we are likely to kick tables, drop cups, and possibly crash cars. Our interpersonal interactions with others during such a day will likely cause us even more irritation, because we are already feeling annoyed, reactive, and easily triggered. The day just gets worse as it progresses.

So why not the opposite possibility? Why do we resist the

idea that we can positively create a *great day* ahead of it happening?

People who meditate at the beginning of every day, or do an hour of yoga, or ride their bike to work, for some examples, will understand that this is effective. They set up their day from the beginning. The events of the day will largely go well, and their day is highly likely to be a smooth and positive series of interactions. Anger doesn't even have a place. *Interactions with other people go smoothly. Gratitude flows. Forgiveness, care, and patience are their key emotions.*

So why do we see this concept as "going soft" or as "unrealistic"? I believe it is because we have collectively held the opposite, negative worldview for so many years. We are surrounded each day by pessimistic outlooks in the conversations we have, the news articles we read or watch on TV, and by our own memories of pain in our earlier lives.

The other reason is that the "tough and resilient" model is still highly regarded in the community and professional groups as being a positive personality attribute, certainly in the medical world.

So, the question to ponder for all of us is how near we are to being ready to make the decision to change. The poem above says it all: *there must be a better way.*

The Journey to Peace

And there is a better way. Getting on our own journeys to peace is **important**. The way ahead is not a solo journey either. The way to our own peace involves a simultaneous endeavour to help the people we are with, or will meet, to find their own type of peace.

In the hospital and ER environment, overcrowding and delays are massive issues. COVID-19 was a big contributor. You would logically think that this environment is the *opposite* of what we need, to generate a sense of inner peace.

And yet it is possible, even in the midst of the craziness, to be a beacon of peace and calm. It all starts with coaxing a tiny flame of peace into being within us. When we do, it feels good. People in the ER comment on the result of this deliberate process often. I really enjoy working shifts with one or two other staff, who are consciously working in a mindful way, generating peace around them as they move through the ER. One of the nurses in particular is also a regular meditator, and she inspires others around her.

We are more effective if we are linked, and several people focusing on inner calm at the same time can have a profound effect, making staff calmer around them and patients more tolerant of delays and the stress of waiting rooms. And behaviour reinforces behaviour, so the effect magnifies further as those calm-creating staff remain focused.

It's all motivated from a place of care.

This shows us up very clearly in a waiting room, when calm receptionists genuinely bring calmness to the waiting patients and family members.

There's no magic to it. We make a decision that we will *deeply care* for all the people—no exceptions—that we will meet in the shift, and we become suitably motivated to do what is required to provide the best of ourselves in that environment.

People always know whether our care for them is genuine or not. They detect our integrity or lack of integrity immediately. So, our job here is to come from real care for others at all times. You have exactly the same skills that I have. We all have it. The only difference is that some of us are conscious of doing this "beacon of peace" thing, and others are still figuring it out.

This idea works—it really, really works. Our mindfulness journey starts at the individual level, and we will quite quickly acquire a few useful things—reduced anxiety, less anger, better sleep patterns, for example—but the next stage is the one we explore *together,* as a collective of humans trying to *achieve something good for others.*

Once we start, we will notice the results in clinical workspaces. Relationships and conversations become golden moments, and our conviction that we are on the right path is further reinforced. Our levels of joy build and build. You will receive feedback from others about the positive impact that you unknowingly had upon their lives, and you will see that as an indication that you are doing what you need to, working from a place of peace, calm and unshakeable mindfulness.

And the best reason is that, as we practice, we start to experience the benefits. We replace pain with peace, which is joy at a deeply resonant level of our being. And that becomes the best reason and the best motivator to *continue* and deepen our journey into mindfulness.

Two of my favourite, somewhat-overused quotes:

1. Mahatma Gandhi: *"Be the change that you wish to see in the world."*

2. Max Ehrmann: *"Go placidly amidst the noise and haste and remember what peace there may be in silence."*

Mindfulness and Scene Control

In an ER resuscitation, we are into "scene control," where we each have clearly defined roles such as 'airway doctor' or 'circulation nurse'. There are protocols for how we treat different conditions, all laid out and logical, and basically, it is the safest way to look after sick patients in a stressful environment.

We need the team in that resuscitation to always be calm and collaborative. We need communication. We certainly need leadership and guidance from the designated team leader.

So, every person in that room needs to understand mindfulness. The inner stillness and outer calm generated by being mindful leads to the resuscitation being a good example of "scene control."

Scene control on an inner level and scene control on an outer level.

The scene control on the inner level creates the scene control on the outer level.

You can see where this is going, of course. By deliberately creating mindfulness internally, we set up our outer world experiences to be calmer, less chaotic, and more cooperative with all the people around us.

And to be completely honest with you, it doesn't *always* go smoothly in the resuscitation room, for various reasons, including the severity of the patient's illness or injuries, or difficulties with interpersonal communications, but it *mostly* does. The aim is to have a mindful resuscitation experience 100 percent of the time.

In other words, once we as individuals start to realise that we can control our inner "emotional weather," we have, from that moment forward, a responsibility to work on our own mindfulness, all the time, and to be role models of that in all our dealings with others.

The change that we are creating within us will affect others around us positively. This is a truth, just as the opposite is a truth—if someone is behaving in an angry way, for example, they can affect others around them in a negative way. I see this sometimes in hospitals, especially in the operating theatre or the ER.

More Reasons…

So, there are **inner** reasons: mindfulness helps us sleep better, feel less indigestion, and generally enjoy more calmness.

There are **interpersonal** reasons: we learn to avoid becoming angry or irritable because we are "tuning up" our skills of self-observation. Our relationships work better, and we like ourselves more.

And then there are the **bigger-picture** reasons: we become a beacon of calm in our workplaces, and we make others calm around us. Conflict lessens. People enjoy working more. They are nicer to their customers.

The funky idea to ponder on, as we close off this chapter, is that these three sets of reasons are all linked together. Very quantum, and very true.

And when we apply unshakeable mindfulness to our lives, we start to learn about a new and durable feeling of resilience that includes *others* and, more importantly, includes those others *in our care*. Strange thing is, the feeling of existential separation from others also fades away. We become the rescuers.

But it starts by *putting on our oxygen mask first*, as they say...

Be the Change

Bless the spaces you work in
Bless the people you are with
Become a beacon of calm
Become a rescuer
Be the change...

A Quick Method to Feel Peace:

Stop moving for a minute or two
Turn off your phone or pager if possible
Close your eyes
Be still and watch your thoughts settle

Stop moving,
maybe sit,
Maybe stand,
Close your eyes,
Let your breathing
be observed.
Now shape your breathing,
slow it down a bit...
Now just watch:
The peaceful feeling comes,
with no effort on your part.
Soak in this silence,
for about a minute,
Go longer if you can.
Then come back to "noise".
But remember how you got here.
The patterns embed as we practice.
We can go back there anytime.

2

NOISE

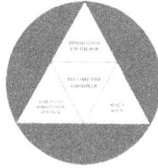

The *unshakeable mindfulness* that we are talking about requires that we can see where we are *starting* from, in order to see the value of making *changes*.

To start to understand inner calm, we start with its opposite, which is *noise*. But let's introduce a child with a developing airway obstruction...

The two-year old boy arrived in the waiting room, stress all over Mum's face as she carried 'James' (not his real name) into ER with a barking cough and severe breathlessness. It was a normal busy Tuesday morning.

Into the resuscitation room, the diagnosis was fairly obvious, even as I scanned through other differentials. Eyes turned towards me as team leader, as oxygen delivery options are gathered. 'James' had acute severe croup, with a high level of accessory muscle usage and work of breathing. The speed of onset had caught James' parents by surprise, compared to several previous milder episodes.

He was getting rapidly worse.

Despite the panic in the little boy himself, who had now become withdrawn and terrified, and the realisation in Mum that something extremely serious was happening, I had to mentally go the other way – into a still place, where I waited for clinical questions, and then answers, to arrive in my mind...

Into that quiet space, ideas and treatment options "came through", and my end-of-bed situational assessment was that we have to turn the situation around quickly. This kid was in trouble, near to respiratory exhaustion from the increased work of breathing.

But from the stillness, the algorithm for our approach became clear. Options for how we would get steroids into him. Positioning him on Mum's lap on the bed. No IV access was needed as yet, but I asked the Procedures Nurse to put on the local anaesthetic patches just in case. I checked the intubation equipment again.

Unshakeable mindfulness. It's like those images of someone on a street who is moving against the crowd, going the other way. It is essential in the ER, especially in a situation like this. The whole team needs it. We take it for granted in our resuscitation team, but there are so many examples of clinical teams that don't operate in such a way, with poor outcomes resulting.

It's easy for our minds to fall into patterns of scattered thinking, or "noise". When we learn techniques of mindfulness or meditation, we learn how to "lower the volume" of this internal noise and return our minds to a place of calm and clarity. Over-writing the noise inside our brains takes practice, a lot of practice, because the "patterns of noise" are ones that we have built up over a long period of time. There is no 5-minute cure for these patterns of thinking and reactivity.

Meditation and mindfulness are all about bringing the scattered thoughts and emotions within our thinking into a calm and focused "laser beam" of more effective thinking, and calmer emotions. It's *unshakeable mindfulness*, because we get strong at insisting on establishing and holding this place in our mind. We don't take any nonsense.

The ideas to follow in these early chapters will examine the challenges of "undoing" the "noise" within our thinking.

"Noise": the Opposite of Calm

Our daily patterns revolve around tension and stress so frequently that we assume it is the *only* way that things can go.

Until we stop, and let stillness return, we may not even be aware of how frenetic and "noisy" our daily lives actually are, especially in the clinical setting. But how many people actually stop the movement, let alone stop their thinking, for a few minutes, or even *one* minute?

A brilliant man once said that *if we keep on doing things the same way, the results will be the same*.

The starting point for learning about stillness is to develop our understanding of its opposite, the concept of *noise.*

Noise is sound that disrupts our other thinking because of its loudness. Noise creates an emotional or even a physical reaction in us. It can be outside us, or inside.

Noise has several levels, and it makes us stressed and tense until we understand it. When we understand mental noise, and how our reactions to that noise are not just random and *out of our control*, we can start to develop a completely new way of reacting to "triggering" people and events around us.

We can't reduce
the noise inside our heads
until we understand
where it comes from.

Noise Comes From Three Sources

1. External noise
2. Internal noise
3. Emotional noise

EXTERNAL   *INTERNAL*

NOISE

EMOTIONAL

External Noise

This means the "out there" noise, not just the noise we hear, but also the constant visual stimulation of TV, screens, and movement all around us, especially in cities.

Stress is caused by all of these types of external noise. A primary example is the *auditory noise* around us, and hospital workplaces are a good example of this noise.

We ER types are surrounded by medical monitors alarming all the time—almost every patient has a blood pressure and cardiac monitor attached during their stay in an emergency department—and alarms ring if the oxygen levels or heart rhythms change.

In other words, in an ER, there's *always* external noise. And coffee.

Noise saturation makes us feel less safe and contributes to background stress. There are physical and psychological effects of stress. Medical errors increase when the environment is noisy and chaotic. Physical noise makes us tense, or it *can,* and affects the emotional environment inside us.

Contrast that with the relative quiet of an operating room team, performing delicate brain surgery. The quietness allows the incredible levels of concentration that are required to bring the patient safely through.

Noise includes loud physical workplaces, airplanes, radio and TV news cycles, and also conversations. Remember also the visual stimulation of screens, streaming services and TV. These are entertainment but are also *noise sources.*

Unless we understand *noise*, it is really hard to understand *silence*.

Most of us spend relatively little time in deliberate silence. Given the choice, if we have a device with a screen nearby and some time to fill, how easily do we default to screen time. The detachment from almost constant audio / visual noise may happen only rarely for a lot of people, and I include myself in this group.

When I finish after a fourteen-hour ER shift, all I want is silence for a time. It's like a reset. Sitting in my car for fifteen minutes of meditation and silence before I go home is sometimes what I really need to do. It makes me saner when I get home to my partner, after the craziness of the working day.

We are frightened of silence; it scares many of us.

Internal Noise

Our *internal noise* could be described as a constant internal discussion going on in the head, flitting between thoughts about the past, the future, and the present moment. We analyse, we judge, we jump ahead, and our minds are kept very busy with the sheer volume of all of these thoughts.

I am a cognitive kind of person. Medical training develops the thinking cognitive parts of us to a large extent. So maybe all medical types are a bit *Type A* like me and tend to "overthink". It's not just seen in doctors, but it certainly does exist in our profession.

The impact of all this *thinking* is that we just never stop doing it. Chatter, more chatter, and then followed by all of the emotional reactions to that chatter. Thinking noise. It is tiring.

The impact of thinking is that we just never stop doing it...

Contrast that with something that involves silence. The ability to touch silence in our minds is in all of us, but it's often a rare experience, unless we go searching for it. However, when we discover the tingling magic of even a moment of profound inner silence, the table tilts, and we realise three things.

Experiencing our first moments of conscious (or even accidental) inner silence teaches us, in a heartbeat, that...

1. There's a much bigger picture going on behind the noise.
2. We have capabilities in us that we never dreamed of.
3. We can grow and develop these abilities.

We all do "accidental silence" moments. Sitting on a beach, being immersed in reading an amazing book, fishing, or doing quiet yoga. For me, a recent example was the inner silence of assembling a swinging seat, studying how the pieces of metal and wood fitted together so precisely, experiencing the simple pleasure of using screwdrivers and spanners, and seeing it all come together. The mental quiet.

Another example was immersing myself in the monotonous task of removing rust and painting a metal beam. It took several sessions, but they were like meditations. So many activities can be used as spontaneous balancing times, or opportunistic meditations – washing dishes, folding clothes, mowing a lawn, or neatly writing up a patient's medical notes, in my case.

Think of some examples of inner silence you have had recently and also of the feeling of those quiet moments.

The opportunities to practice these new skills are all around us. The high-level practice opportunities come when we are learning a new way of reacting to "triggers", and we will discuss this in Chapter 6.

We could define *internal noise* as a continuous rolling of a film; a constant projection of characters, plot twists and story-lines. A collection of neurons always firing and creating traffic of the mind, even while we are asleep.

Our brains have so much noise in them for large parts of every minute, every hour, and every day.

There has to be a better way of thinking.

Internal thinking noise is also overlaid with our *emotional reactions* to each of those thoughts, like a spiderweb.

Our thoughts have favourite *themes*, for example, a situation or relationship issue that is worrying us, or a nagging feeling that we are not good enough in some way. Our thinking cycles back to narratives within each theme, and the episodes of thinking about that particular narrative are often repetitive and similar in content.

Commonly, there will be an attached emotional thread, meaning that we may be thinking something like "I am no good; I don't deserve this job/position/relationship," in response to that particular thought.

In our untrained mind, the emotional reaction (or even a physical reaction, like a racing heart or sweating with sudden anxiety) seems to be a completely involuntary or automatic process that is *triggered* by the thinking content. As if we have no control over it.

But there's the third kind of noise.

Emotional Noise

We all have different intrinsic emotional patterns. We call this our intrinsic personality, and our patterns are unique to each of us. These patterns are determined or influenced by our upbringing, our family experiences, and what we have learnt to be useful behaviours for our professional or home roles. Doctors are trained to be non-reactive and to behave calmly under pressure, for example, but that is *not* always an indication of mindfulness or a genuine feeling of calm within. It is certainly not "unshakeable mindfulness".

Of course, this is a medical stereotype, but it is also an

example of how we all have internal patterns of emotional reaction. And we can change this.

In fact, some of us are the *complete* opposite to the medical stereotype described above. Reactive to everything.

We see in the hospital setting how some senior doctors react to any delays, or to not having everything ready - other staff creep around them so as not to wake the 'angry bear'. This is toxic at every level of a workplace, and in the individual as well. Health worries, the tiring effect of stress or anger—none of it is good.

Can We Change?

Yes. We can reach *unshakeable mindfulness*. Effectively and quickly.

So, there is noise coming at us from these three levels, which are

1. Outside us;
2. Inside us - our thoughts; and
3. Inside us - our emotional reactions.

But let's just simplify this and call it the collective "noise".

Simply observing the noise makes it go quiet .

Mindfulness is just a modern description for a state of mind that enables us to quieten noise in our thinking and emotions. *Meditation* is an important mind-training strategy with many related techniques. There are many styles, but let's keep it simple.

We learn to *observe the noise* in our thinking and emotional reactions, and then to choose another way. And make it unshakeable.

The first step toward rescuing ourselves from a feeling of constant stress is to acknowledge the problem for what it is. By observing the myriad ways that we generate internal noise, and our stressful reactions to external events, we can begin the process of inner change.

Simply observing the noise makes it go quiet. If we become unshakeable observers of our own patterns, we take back control of the pattern. This is *unshakeable mindfulness* in action.

- Mindfulness training is all about learning how to observe the moment we are in *right now*.
- If we focus on being good observers, our brain has no spare bandwidth to generate noise, anxiety, and stress.
- We *can* only concentrate on one thing at a time.
- Becoming incredibly determined to achieve this creates *unshakeable mindfulness*.

Over some anxious hours, James finally responded to much higher doses of nebulised adrenaline and steroids than we usually need to use. He did not require intubation and ventilation. Unshakeable mindfulness was crucial to the process of observing

him closely, weighing up the various options and waiting for the
eventual improvement.

Let's break this thing wide open, let's look at change, and
move on to look at the concept of Silence.

Activity:

A "**5-breath-meditation**" practice:

> Eyes open: take **one** breath in and out, slowly
> Eyes closed: take **one** breath, in and out, slowly
> Eyes open: take **two** breaths in and out, slowly
> Eyes closed: take **two** breaths, in and out, slowly
> Eyes open: take **three** breaths in and out, slowly
> Eyes closed: take **three** breaths, in and out, slowly
> Eyes open: take **four** breaths in and out, slowly
> Eyes closed: take **four** breaths, in and out, slowly
> Eyes open: take **five** breaths in and out, slowly
> Eyes closed: take **five** breaths, in and out, slowly

This kind of mindfulness exercise may be unfamiliar because
we are more used to *doing* rather than being *quiet*.

Tips for Setting up an Unshakeable and Mindful Day

- Try this: set your wake-up time 15 minutes earlier.
- Get up and sit to practice meditation (the 5-breath-
  meditation above is one example, or see suggestions
  in the next chapter, "Silence").
- Do it for 15 minutes.
- If 15 minutes is too long, try 5 minutes.

This is a transition practice from 'busy thoughts' to 'calm thoughts' that shows that integrating some basic mindfulness meditation into your schedule does <u>not</u> have to be hard to do.

3

SILENCE

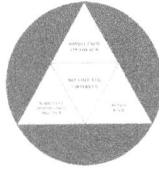

It was a normal busy Friday evening and the 17-year-old young woman, let's call her Heidi, had gotten in the way of a thrown beer glass at a local bar. She had been drinking but was able to recall events. Heidi had blood down her face from two significant lacerations, one a deep 2cm (3/4 inch) cut across the bridge of her nose, and the other a 4cm (1.5 inch) diagonal sloping gash across her left eyebrow. There was no plastic surgeon cover available, so it was up to me to fix it.

The usual questions emerge, establishing whether she had glass in her eye, or any visual injury. Did she lose consciousness? No scans were needed fortunately. Explaining to her, and her worried parents, that I would need to carefully explore the wounds after injecting a long-acting local anaesthetic. Telling them how any small clear glass fragments in either wound, would need to be removed before starting the slow process of putting the skin edges back together and adjusting the levels to line up the wound layers, using tiny stitches and the magnifying lenses.

To do this, I needed to reach the now-familiar place of concentration and silence, and remain there, while I could take in all the elements of the wound and how the repair would need to be achieved. The conversations with Heidi and her parents would cease during the procedure – it required silence, externally and internally.

Addressing the Pattern...

During the busiest parts of a shift in the ER at the hospital, I will notice my mind flying around, often in random directions, from thought to thought. There may be an associated *feeling* with those thoughts, which is the *emotional noise* that we talked about in Chapter 2. Our untrained mind generates so much mental and emotional clutter.

Our reactions to conversations, our decisions, and our subsequent actions are really important. Making decisions from a place of noise and stress is not our strongest strategy. This is what we commonly mean when we say of someone who is easily triggered, "Oh, he's just a very reactive kind of person."

Making decisions from a place of noise and stress is not our strongest strategy.

In hospitals, we certainly have people like that, and their ability to care for patients or colleagues is compromised because of the *emotional noise* level within the doctor, nurse, or clerk involved. Sometimes, those staff need mentoring, or even to be moved elsewhere to protect the all-important *culture of care* in the ER.

We've all got different set-points. Some of us are naturally fairly calm, but others of us are highly reactive. But contrary to what we are told, our minds are *not* set in concrete, in terms of this *inherent reactivity*. Mindfulness defines this set-point as our *default pattern*, and we can change it with practice.

But we may initially assume that we *can't* change these reaction patterns. Going back a step, the first part of the problem is that we don't even *observe* our own patterns of reacting. We just barrel on, reacting as we have always done. Throwing emotional hand grenades around unknowingly, hurting ourselves, others, and our relationships. The idea that we *can* observe ourselves is a bit radical, but it is the start-point of mindfulness training.

But it Requires Work

The journey of change simply won't happen until we do that.

In emergency departments, we are usually Type A personalities and fairly action-based. Reflection and contemplation is not an easy "fit" with the constant activity of the job. It may happen for brief moments, for example when we are waiting in the coffee line at the hospital cafeteria.

Changing our patterns takes work. Listening to a meditation podcast or flipping through that self-help book in the shelves of a bookshop won't get us there. A lot of self-help journeys start and fizzle, simply because we can't keep on with the discipline of daily practice.

Strange as it seems, our *natural* way is calmness and flow. However, our natural pattern is buried *underneath* our stress reaction and thinking patterns. Given half a chance, usually in the form of a few days of holiday, perhaps in the wilderness or by a beach, our natural patterns re-emerge, and we start to think in a more relaxed and happier way again. Instinctively, we know when we "need to take a break", because we are magnetically drawn to calm.

Observing the problem is the very first step.

But as most of us also know, we can *undo* the positive effects of a holiday within a day or so of returning to our usual activities! In other words, our trained and habitual reaction patterns set back in, and we are back in stress, wondering why we even went on the holiday in the first place.

We each carry many habitual patterns of thinking and reacting to situations or triggers. Most of these create stress, and some create conflict or anger when we bring them out for yet another "re-run".

It takes discipline to turn this ship around.

We need to do whatever it takes to discard the thinking patterns that are counter-productive. As we do, we will reach a state of calmness, infrequently at first, but more and more often as we practice. The really good news is that it gets easier and faster to flick across from stress to calm.

From that perhaps unfamiliar state of calm, all sorts of transformations can then occur in our health and in our relationships.

The first step is to quantify the problem – to run some "diagnostic tests" – and from there we can look at developing our strategy for change – or "selecting the correct treatment", to use medical terminology.

We talked earlier of becoming our own observer, watching our stress reactions, and watching how we respond immediately to "triggers" in the environment.

Let's look at the transition from stress to calm, as they tentatively look at mindfulness and meditation.

It's the most common stage for people to experience difficulty...

From Stress to Calm...

Let's start by conceptualising the stages of thinking as we go from **stress** to **calm**:

1. **Normal Thought:** our daily life, typical busy thinking

2. **Early Stages:** we sit, we close our eyes, we stop moving around

3. **Deep Calm**: slowing, spacious thinking, as we approach stillness

Normal Thought

Our waking minds are, for the most part, a mix of disorganised thoughts, emotions, and some productive ideas. Our thoughts help us with achieving tasks and transferring ideas to other people, but there is a lot of peripheral mental activity associated.

"Normal Thought" is such a familiar place for us to be in that we have no idea that it is *not* our natural state. Most of us believe that it represents the *whole* picture of how our mind works. Furthermore, we may believe that we have *no control over it*.

This pattern is reinforced each day, as we go through the day, and react in the same way. Our brain actively resists any change in the status quo. We each have our patterns of thinking and interpreting the world around us, with resulting emotional reaction patterns that are predictable, as our brain keeps on falling into the same reaction habits, time after time.

Sooner or later, we have to change...

And we will eventually realise, that something has to give. Perhaps it's a crunch or crisis, or a major relationship falling apart, or just deciding that the grinding stress of our life is intolerable. I think that one key reason many people give up on meditation / mindfulness is that they find the transition process away from Normal Thought *so hard*. It is, at first, because our mind hates the discipline of becoming still, or even of observing what is actually going on with our thoughts. But the solution starts with observing the problem, as someone once wrote.

Mastering Normal Thought - Practice Makes Perfect

Distrust anyone who says that you can master meditation or mindfulness with a single retreat, or their 5-week online course. You *can* pick up the beginnings of the knowledge and techniques of meditation, but real progress comes from repetition. Teaching our minds to think and react differently takes regular practice.

Medical students have to learn procedures, such as suturing wounds, inserting IV drips into patient's veins, and progressively, as they become full doctors, more advanced procedures including surgery and managing patients with severe trauma, such as motor vehicle crashes or serious wounds.

When we teach junior staff a procedural skill, we have to break it down into easy sections. And we may have to go over the lesson many times. "Wash your hands", "put on gloves", "open up the sterile field", etc.

Meditation is the same in the early stages. Initially, meditation seems intellectual, but even with a few practice sessions we will experience its benefits.

The idea of even closing our eyes, and sitting quietly, is a very uncomfortable concept for some people, especially those with severe anxiety disorders, or a life experience that makes it hard for them to trust others. They feel as if they need to always be "on guard" for threats of various kinds. We see this in returned soldiers who have PTSD after their military experiences.

As we progress, the intellectual ideas are replaced more and more by the *feeling* of calmness. It becomes something that we really want. We will each discover our own unique experiences - and some common ones - as we progress into the vast world of meditation.

And Another Thing

Keeping to a daily meditation discipline is a way of saying to ourselves that this short time commitment is *important*:

- Important for our well-being,
- Important for "setting up the day ahead", and
- Important for the outcomes of any interactions with others.

Early Stages

When we sit down to practice silence and close our eyes, we go from the day-to-day "Normal Thought" into an *intermediate* phase of mindfulness / meditation which I will call "Early Stages". The names don't matter as such, but they help convey the concept that there is a linear transition from fully activated thinking, down to "Deep Calm" thinking. However, the real understanding starts when we begin our mindfulness and meditation practice.

As we start a mindfulness practice session, by closing our eyes, we immediately and significantly reduce external sensory stimuli, but often our mind, which is so well trained in the intellectual domain, continues to fire away in the form or thoughts, emotional reactions or physiological reactions.

Yet as we continue to sit, our thoughts will quite naturally slow, a bit like dust settling.

Two things happen when we close our eyes. If we are lying down or in a comfortable chair, we can fall asleep. This is probably why most meditation traditions don't recommend starting off our practice by lying down. The meditation morphs into *sleep*.

This is not harmful in any way, and we may sleep better for it, but it isn't meditation. It is sleep, and there *are* times when our body and mind are so tired from the day's events that meditation is impossible. At those moments, we probably just need to get some sleep. On the other hand, people are often drawn to explore meditation because they experience high levels of anxiety and *cannot* sleep.

In those Early Stages practice sessions, we may sit there feeling a little embarrassed, knowing that this mindfulness stuff is supposed to be therapeutic and good for us, but the shopping lists and worries just keep on scrolling down our inner mental screen, like the green lines of scrolling digits in the Matrix films.

And yet this is perfectly OK and does not mean that we are failures at meditation. Rome wasn't built in a day and all that. It is *repetition* that helps us break through. We lose our calmness, and then we return to the breathing exercise, or the mantra word, or the body scan – whatever approach we are using to slowly build our concentration. Concentration leads to calm.

Concentration leads to calm.

This can be a frustrating stage when many beginners declare that they *just can't meditate*. And understandably enough, they stop altogether. Just as I did, for some years.

Even now, as a daily meditator, I still get pulled into distracting thoughts when I am meditating, and have to apply the strategies in this book to dig myself out, to stop the world of the Normal Thought. The distracting thoughts are normal, and once we recognise them, we can pull ourselves back on track *quickly*, with a few techniques that work. The 5-breath-meditation described above is one such powerful method that I have tested in my medical students with success.

Another way of seeing the Normal Thought → Early Stages → Deep Calm transition is the analogy of running into the sea to go surfing. The most difficult water to cross is the first part, with choppy waves and no real speed as yet, to help us move through or over the waves.

The transition period described above initially feels *vibratory* and *shaky*, but it fades, and I see it as just another obstacle that our overactive Normal Thought brains throw up to test our resolve. It settles with determined practice.

The initial destination in meditation is Deep Calm, which

feels as if our thinking is becoming very slow and spacious. Verbal thinking speed seems to *slow down*.

We have all reached Deep Calm spontaneously, for example when we are watching a beach sunset with someone special, or when the fishing is relaxing us completely, or when we are jogging comfortably and feeling in the zone - there are so many examples. Time spent in Deep Calm heals us, we love it. It is addictive once we experience it. It *is* our natural state of being. Our brain has things the wrong way round, believing that our natural state of being is Normal Thought. Stress does us so much harm, and negatively affects our relationships with ourselves, others, and the world around us. Normal Thought is based on swirling emotion, mostly negative, and often self-undermining. It can also be about feelings of attack or being attacked.

Expanding a Calm Space

So how do we change our *default pattern* of reacting and thinking, the bouncing of random mental clutter and the associated emotional and bodily stress reactions?

By quietly expanding a calm space at the centre of the noise, we break up the trajectories of those thoughts. Imagine an old-time Main Street gunfight in a Western movie, with shots being fired from hidden windows in every building on the street. Then imagine dumping fifty tons of sand right in the middle of the street. The gunfighters can't shoot through the sand, so the exchange of bullets loses its momentum.

We can use mental strategies in a similar way, to *break up the thoughts*. One strategy might work, for example a relaxation breathing technique, which is great. But often, our intellectual minds distract us to draw us back to Normal Thought, so we need to have a few other options ready to use.

In other words, all of the techniques I will describe are intended to build our concentration, by breaking up the familiar and frenetic *thinking patterns* that most of us spend our lives in every day.

This breaking up of the thinking patterns is Deep Calm. It is the start of real experience in a meditation session.

So how do we reach this, and for Type A doctors like me, how do we achieve this *efficiently and reliably*?

Firstly, *don't worry* about whether or not you reach any stage. Just do the practice – breathing, mantra, slow walking, yoga, a hobby - whatever you choose. The repetition takes care of the rest.

Practising the transition is *not* easy, especially at first, but it *becomes* easy with practice. Our waking thinking mind resists silence, at first. And then Deep Calm becomes a launch platform for going further and further into meditative states.

In the early transition zones (Normal Thought and Early Stages), language is crucial, a bit like directions on a treasure map. One of the many learnings in meditation is that our minds can operate in meditation *without* language. Meditation is more of a *feeling* thing. And yes, it is hard to explain in words!

Sure, we need language for day-to-day living and communication, but there are many, many levels at which our mind can work, and the further reaches of the journey are more accurately described in *feelings* rather than *language*. And from these levels of other experience, we bring back an unfamiliar sense of calm, clarity, and purpose to our day-to-day world.

All of the great meditation traditions were developed by people who understood the crazy ways that our brains operate and think. The various strategies have the same outcome, which is to help us centre and *stop the mental chatter* of our minds, in other words, to achieve a breakthrough *quietness* within the Normal Thought world. The Buddhists have a term called "monkey mind" to describe the "noise" that we explored in Chapter 2. It's a good analogy.

We can see our mind as a mobile spotlight where *we* are the controller of the light. We can choose what we see, what we focus on, and *how we react to what we see.*

If we practice simple repetitive sequences, and choose to focus on those, we will effectively quieten our Normal Thought.

Unshakeable mindfulness is when we know the methods that work for us, and whenever we recognise the need to re-balance, we *apply* them. Either during scheduled daily practice sessions, or *immediately.* No questions asked. We apply the methods, and we get the positive results that we want.

Let's look at how we build concentration, to reach towards calm. We will look at two tried and trusted meditation techniques, the first one is *breathing*, the second one involves slow internal repetition of a word, also known in meditation as a *mantra...*

Technique 1: Breathing

Breathing is the classic example. We all breathe and are barely aware of breathing. Which is just as well, as we churn through our working days, when we need focus for outside activities, conversations, etc.

But in meditation, breathing is something we can pay conscious attention to. As we practice, our concentration on our breathing becomes unshakeable. We just learn how to focus on our breathing. It is deceptively simple, yet so very hard, especially as we start along this path called *mindfulness.*

But it is worth the effort, even at the beginner's level, when we lose our concentration often. The process of focus, or concentrating on something, effects positive change. Our thoughts start to synchronise, like photons in a laser. We become calm.

There is no need to try and *control* the breathing, apart from just observing the pattern of our breathing as it naturally becomes slower and smoother. At Deep Calm levels, our breathing becomes very slow, sometimes there is a pause between breaths, and at other times we may take a couple of quicker shallow breaths. It all becomes very still. Without forcing, without worrying about results or achieving.

If you do your own research, you will see mindfulness and meditation articles describing the square breathing pattern or counting to different numbers on the in-breaths, followed by a brief pause, then letting the breath out slowly.

There are many patterns, none any better than the others, and with the same outcome. Breath observation is a proven technique for crossing the Normal Thought → Deep Calm transition, but it is not the only one.

As we meditate it is normal to switch back and forth between the states of Early Stages ←→ Deep Calm ←→ Early Stages. This is not a problem. We all do it.

With regular practice, transition times to Deep Calm decrease (to several seconds or even *immediately* when closing one's eyes), and the time we can sustain in Deep Calm expands, with less and less effort. Time spent in the Deep Calm phase seems to be the main ingredient for then easily moving to even deeper levels of relaxation.

We can measure these scientifically. The phases of meditation correlate with brain activity on EEG tracings (electroencephalograph or brain wave measuring machines). It's possible to measure and watch meditators transitioning from waking *beta* brain wave frequency (fourteen to twenty-one electrical cycles per second), down into relaxation *alpha* frequency (seven to fourteen cycles per second), and on into deep relaxation or *theta* frequency (four to seven cycles per second).

For the scientists who are researching meditation, these are objective measures of the ability of a meditator to *transition*, as in the **Normal Thought / Early Stages / Deep Calm** transitions that we are talking about. As well as detecting change of phase, when the brain wave frequency changes abruptly, we can approximately confirm that a meditator is in either a *light* meditation or alternatively a *deep* meditation.

But is this really helpful at an individual experiential level of mindfulness?

I suppose that we *could* wire ourselves up to an EEG and use it as a biofeedback comparison tool to help with meditation. There are also effective music tracks widely available that incorporate certain frequency metronome beats inside relaxing music tracks, and they are useful in the early stages for some people as tools to facilitate phase transition from Early Stages to Deep Calm.

After the early stages of getting used to the discipline of meditation, we just don't need the accessories. By *accessories*, I mean meditation music, guided meditation scenarios, metronomes at brainwave frequencies, or meditation glasses with flashing LEDs. All of these devices *will* influence our brain frequencies toward the meditative levels, but they will eventually become a distraction and unnecessary. All we need is the silence, which we are becoming better and better at generating, within our thinking.

Technique 2: Mantra

Another of the different options for disrupting the Normal Thought thinking is the use of *mantras*, which are basically words that we speak silently to ourselves during meditation, every few seconds. Link the word repetitions to the cycle of your breathing. By concentrating on the sound or rhythm of the mantra, we disrupt our day-to-day thinking. That same phrase, *concentration leads to calm*.

A mantra can be any word or phrase that we want to use. The sound of the word alone is enough; for example, we are all familiar with the images of meditators speaking mantra words aloud as they meditate, classically something like "Om," but any word or sound has an effect.

Some mantras are intense words, like "Love" or "God" or "Peace." But we don't have to use these words. In certain meditation traditions, the mantra provided to a meditation student is a Sanskrit word that means little to us. "God" or "Om" or other religious words have enormous power for some people and will form an integral part of their meditation or prayer practice. These words will not resonate with others.

"Love" or "Peace" or other inspiring words will work better for others. We could choose to *exclude* words with spiritual connotations, or just choose something like "Calm". Using *any* word repetitively imbues that word with special meaning, for us.

Just repeat your chosen word very quietly every few seconds, so as not to disrupt the Deep Calm feeling as it naturally develops.

If you get distracted, and we all do, quietly bring your attention back to the mantra. It gets easier. But don't try with the aim of maintaining concentration for 20 minutes. Start with 2 minutes perhaps, or 5 minutes. Be realistic.

Where's This All Going?

Breathing exercises and mantra repetitions are just two tried and tested examples of meditation techniques that build our concentration, by developing effective and rapid mental and bodily stillness.

At its core, meditation is about *disrupting the thinking patterns* that aren't helping us anymore. Maybe they never helped us. Perhaps they were useful for a few years, but now we sense that they aren't working.

So, we are training our mind to *disrupt these patterns deliberately* by developing strategies that work. Breathing is a proven and powerful meditation technique, and mantras are effective also, to distract our mind from dwelling on all the noise in our lives. That's the basis for reaching unshakeable mindfulness.

Later, we will take a deeper dive into other concepts of escaping from our current patterns of thinking and reacting.

Back to the ER Scenario...

As I cleaned, injected local anaesthetic, and studied how the wound must have been created, the map of how it could be put back together emerged. A part of my mind was thinking about the cosmetic implications for Heidi, as both wounds were in prominent and visible areas of her face.

Technical aspects came through with questions – will I use the 5-0 or the 6-0 suture thread. Are the magnifying lenses in focus? Will I use adrenaline with the local anaesthetic on her eyebrow? Was that a clink of a glass fragment in the wound, and where is it now?

A 3-dimensional map of how it would come together was forming, along with the placement of the stitches I would place...

The wound repair was finally complete. Cleaning, drying and applying dressings. After giving advice for wound care and removal of sutures, Heidi and her parents were on their way home. Then on to the next patient.

Activity:

- Sit down and arrange your limbs comfortably.
- As you settle your breathing slowly, start to repeat your word or mantra,
- Think the word in coordination with your breathing.

For example, we could choose the word "thankyou". So, as you breathe in slowly, mentally say "thank you". After that breath, say another "thank you", as you start to breathe out.

Keep on doing it:
Breathe in.
"Thank you."
Breathe out.
"Thank you."
...and so on.

Gradually, your thinking will slow.
Your breathing will become calm
A few minutes may be enough,
at the Deep Calm level.
Or continue for longer,
if you feel comfortable.
Then, gradually, *come back*,
Perhaps with some slow muscle-stretching,
as you return to Normal Thought level...
Open your eyes when you are ready.

- Daily practice periods of such techniques develop our capability to "spin down" rapidly.
- With frequent sessions, the Normal Thought to Deep Calm transitions become automatic, and *fast*.
- It all becomes reliable, something to be *trusted*.

4

SKILLS

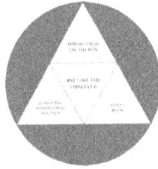

This day in ER was already crazy – a blur of moving doctors and nurses as we criss-crossed the work areas, patients coming in, onto beds, beds emptying as the patients were rolled across the corridor to have the all-important CT scans or ultrasounds.

Information. It's all information. Each piece helps put the diagnosis together. And then we need to look at other possibilities. There's a list of "make sure" questions that we must ask. We call them the "safety questions".

To ask these safety questions, we need to be quite still for a few minutes in our mind. If we can find that stillness, even for a short time, the questions will find the answers that help to keep our patients safe.

It's easy on a mindfulness retreat to be calm. It's easy halfway through a holiday to feel relaxed. But in the ER, the noise drives calm away.

It's what we mean by an unshakeable mindfulness. It's two things: firstly, a recognition of the chaos and continual noise of modern emergency departments, and secondly, a determination that nothing will distract me from finding the stillness that allows thinking, searching through the incoming information. Searching, and then finding. Finding the diagnosis that saves a life.

...my next patient was a 94-year-old man, who had tripped over his walking frame. It can happen so easily. A fall onto his wrist, hitting his head on the way down the door frame. He was complaining of severe pain and bruising in his wrist. There was also a bleeding laceration along the thin forearm, and so the nurses applied a temporary dressing to stop the bleeding. I thought he would need some stitches and probably a plaster, after we had some X-Rays done...

One of my junior doctors comes with me when we first assess each new patient. I start by asking a few key questions, then we discuss our initial impressions of what we think is going on, and I suggest a list of imaging investigations and blood tests. "Are you OK with doing those things?", I ask as I delegate to the young trainee and move on to see the next patient.

The calmness has to hold. So many patients, so few beds at times, and always the intensity that severe illness can create. Low blood pressure, any change in conscious state, a sudden high pulse rate or a rising fever. It's continuous multi-tasking and it's all important to get right.

So that's the situation I work in each day, and *why* I need an unshakeable mindfulness. And I reach this "place" again by sending some quieting thoughts internally, some thoughts of profound reassurance, and by observing and taking several very slow breaths. The old "take three deep breaths" routine, even while walking through the ER to the next patient.

But it's much more effective if we understand some basic skills, because like all skills, it's not so much the initial learning of something, but the repetition to really *drum it in*...

The Journey So Far

In Chapter 2, we looked at *noise* and how we surround ourselves with inner and outer noise, comprising our thoughts about what is happening *around* us and *to* us, as well as the noise of our emotional reactions to these events.

Most of Us Assume This is Normal

Then, in Chapter 3, we introduced the concept of *turning down the noise*. In mindfulness terminology they call this *changing our default pattern* of reactions to everything going on. We recognised three levels of this process, beginning at "Normal Thought", then through "Early Stages", and down to "Deep Calm".

It's not the labels that matter, but grasping the general concept –

We CAN change our patterns of thinking and reacting, especially the ones that hurt.

Calmness in *any* situation, (which we keep on describing, for a very good reason, as **unshakeable mindfulness**) and more effective relationships, are the potential benefits from consciously developing skills in transitioning down from *Normal Thought* to *Deep Calm*.

We started to look at some ways that we can alter our reactions to events and thoughts, introducing simple techniques borrowed from mindfulness and meditation, which can enable us to step outside our default reaction patterns.

In clinical medicine, we have this concept called "teaching on the run", which is all about devising creative teaching methods for quick tutorials in busy workplaces, such as the ER.

In a way, all the short and quick meditation techniques in this book are a bit like that; we are teaching our brains new patterns of reacting and thinking, to remember and apply as we go through the "normal" busy day of activity...

This practice of "watching air move" sounds simple enough, right? Let's expand on this. We are all familiar with getting caught up in the traffic of our minds. By stepping out of the traffic, and becoming the observer through mindful breathing, you find *stillness*. Eventually, you will be able to do this in a crowded room. I am at the point now where I can do this mindful breathing exercise intermittently through the ER shift, in those moments when I am not actually in a conversation. Also, another favourite stillness and breathing practice is while I wait to pick up a coffee order for the ER nurses and doctors. We can all do this.

This exercise is not intended for the perfect quiet conditions of a meditation studio, complete with tinkling chimes and bamboo forest scenes. It is intended for the hustle of daily life. Your daily life. My daily life.

Keeping your eyes open and fairly still, while looking at something, works well for meditating in public spaces. Meditating on trains and buses is easy, or while walking, but is not recommended for safety reasons while driving or crossing a road.

Each activity in this book is designed to be simple, and to become easier still as we try each one out a few times.

The meditation (aka mindfulness) techniques we will explore can be split into some "on the run" strategies, and others for use in "longer sessions" of practice.

Scheduling Practice:
Many meditation students
schedule their practice
at the beginning of the day,
just after waking up,
but last thing at night works also.
Having less distractions helps.

Meditation "On the Run"

This is funky stuff because most people around us may not be consciously aware that we are doing micro-meditations throughout our working day.

But they will notice that there is something different about you, particularly as you apply these practices over a period of time.

Meditators become less combustible, less irritable, consistently happier, and a force for good in their family, workplace, or social group. You will definitely be noticed.

So, let's describe some techniques that work in the middle of the noise of the average day.

They say that emergency doctors have a short attention span, and this is certainly true. So, we will start with a summary...

"Meditation on the run" can be understood using the four characteristics shown below.

1. Breath
2. Movement
3. Focus
4. Care

Breath

The breathing activities we have described so far may have been new to some. The process of observing changes things. Even just watching our breathing, as we did above, has a measurable effect on reducing the noise levels in our head. Our brain's electricity starts to become quieter, and we notice the difference. And it is cumulative. Next time we do this, we reach even *greater* levels of stillness quite rapidly. Try it. Even for a minute, while you stir your coffee perhaps.

Our mind needs discipline. I don't mean the kind that we see in classrooms or in basic military training. We have this cacophony of noise going on in the Normal Thought. Yet most of us at some level, have an unexpressed longing for *more peace*.

Why do we use breathing? There are several reasons. Breathing gives us an instant *read* on what is going on with our thinking and emotions. Hyperventilation during panic attacks is an extreme example of this.

Making Our Breathing Work for Us

We have shown that just observing our breathing starts to calm us. It's not always easy to recall this technique when we feel overwhelmed or tense. But repetition changes habit, so we all must start somewhere. Celebrate even the *first* time that you try this during a stressful moment. Next time will be even *more* effective.

Breathing exercises involve **imagination**, and using two strategies at once makes the calming effect much more effective. In other words, if we do a breathing exercise to restore calm and imagine the breath going out, then coming back in toward us, we occupy more parts of our mind that otherwise would be going into stress mode. By keeping our mind busy, the stress loses its grip, even if just a little at first.

As our breathing slows, by using observation, perhaps with a simple visualisation added, as in the above example, we can shape our breathing into an even more relaxed cycle and build an even greater degree of calmness.

As we concentrate on the breathing exercise, the noisy thoughts quieten, because we are not giving our attention to them.

Movement

We can see now that observing breathing creates a space for enabling Normal Thought to Deep Calm transitions. We can further accelerate this *slowing down* process by adding mental imagery that we associate with quietness, and by doing this, we *distract* our busy mind. Strange as it may seem, calmness is actually our *true* default state.

We are the ones who create the stress, the emotion, and the feelings of separation.

But we are not there yet. It takes consistent work to loosen the grappling hooks. Initially, all of this calmness stuff feels impossible and unrealistic. But by practicing the techniques here - or any other techniques from mindfulness or relaxation training - we can create a space for our mind to be open to the *possibility of change,* and by practicing whenever we can through the day, even for a few seconds, we can *remind ourselves* of that.

So, for me, I use any activity I can to calm the mind through focus and attention to the meditative process. For example, I use deliberate and smooth movements to reduce my stress levels when I am putting on a plaster cast or suturing a wound back together – as in the example at the start of this chapter...

In each activity, I concentrate on the smoothness of the movement, as I tie a knot with deliberate flowing movements of my hands or smooth the wet plaster cast on someone's broken wrist. And I watch my breathing as I do it. These very medical activities can be achieved in a very Zen way and I believe that the end result is of more benefit to the patient, if I use this approach.

Also, when writing an X-ray referral, I try to make the letters smooth and flowing, a bit like calligraphy. The process of creating the letters brings my mind from noise to quietness, even for a few seconds.

Each strategy starts to blur into the others as we practice meditation. As we slow our breathing or just observe it, our breathing will fall into step, and become calmer. Similarly, with movement meditation we are just using deliberate and slow body movement to bring a feeling of calm to our thoughts and emotional reactions.

The end result is that you *will* master all of this, and eventually break through to a less stressed way of moving through your busy life.

Focus

A Catholic nun once said to me,*"Whenever you enter a room, send a blessing to that space."*

And she was right. I watched her once as she walked around the hospital, visiting every patient to speak some kind and encouraging words. She would even stop briefly in empty rooms, to say a short prayer before moving on.

It took me twenty years to figure out what she was doing.

To her words, I would add the following, *"And send a blessing to all who you will meet in that space."*

If the word "blessing" is uncomfortable for you, then simply change it to something like "sending your good will" or "sending kind thoughts." The general theme of meditation is that *you* create the language and terminology that feels right for you.

So why is this useful? What has it got to do with mindfulness? And why am I emphasising this as important?

As with many things, an idea is often taught by looking at its opposite. Let's look at the opposite. Imagine instead going into a room, carrying with you a cloud of irritation, just wanting to be *anywhere* else but there. The day has started badly, you got out on the wrong side of the bed... we have all done this.

If you let yourself be angry, and it is a *choice* you make at some level, it is highly likely that you will encounter anger as you progress through your day. It is likely that you will bump into things, or scratch your car in the parking lot, or even make errors as you do your work.

In the ER, errors are incredibly serious, and angry doctors are high risk for the staff and patients around them, to the extent that they often cannot be allowed to stay working in the ER.

The *opposite* situation is generated by sending a blessing to the spaces we go into.

Let's See Why it Works...

By sending the blessing, we are sending out *care* to others, whoever they might be. We are regaining control over any irritation we might be feeling, and sending our inner selves a strong message that we are *not* going to let triggers around us create negative emotional reactions in us. We are setting ourselves up for success.

In emergency medicine, we call this *a culture of clinical safety.* It's probably obvious by now that a calm senior doctor in a resuscitation situation is the one you would want looking after you or your loved ones.

Calm leaders create calm in the people near them.

They instil confidence, and actively invite contributions and ideas from others in the room. They build trust, and the patients do better. A great ER "safety culture" is the result.

So we can see how starting our day with such a focus or giving the blessing, as my nun friend did, with such simplicity and devotion, is genuinely helpful to our state of mind.

And if we add *focus* to *breath* and *movement* in combination, the results are indeed powerful. Powerful for ourselves, but more importantly in a clinical situation, powerful for others around us.

And this brings me to the point where I get *off* the "mindfulness bus." Because a lot of self-help strategies are very self-focused. By its nature, the "self-help movement" can be inherently *individualistic*, as if the answers to our human dilemmas can arise in *isolation* from our fellow travellers.

So, our fastest progress in all of this comes when we finally realise that it is *not* about us. It's all about our responsibility as medical professionals to care for others.

Care

Because ER doctors and nurses must do shift handovers every few hours to the incoming staff, we get plenty of practice at summarising. So here is one, in case you missed it.

Several techniques can be used in isolation to reduce our stress levels. These include the many *breath* techniques developed through the years in martial arts, tai chi, and yoga. I have described the next group of these stillness transition strategies under the heading of *movement*. Finally, the deliberate decision to set up each day and each moment in an uncompromisingly mindful way, I have called *focus*.

The combination of all of these gives momentum to our quest. But the final strategy is deciding it's all really important.

We all know the story: "Yeah, I tried meditation and mindfulness, but I couldn't stick at it?", or, "It was really boring, actually."

To overcome that distractibility, we can develop a range of options which we can use either singly or in combination.

But bringing all of these meditation strategies together, using bits of one or bits of another scattered throughout our day, is transformative. And when we dedicate all of every day to this process, not just for us, but for the people around us, we really accelerate. That's what I mean by "care".

Activity 1:

Breathing and Mental Imagery

As you do your breathing practice, bring up the image of someone casting a fishing line onto the smooth surface of a lake. The way that they lay the line flat on the water, with hardly a ripple, and then they wind the line back in. It is hypnotic to watch.

Now on each "out breath," imagine your breath casting out in the same effortless manner, and on the "in breath," imagine winding the line quickly in.

Each sequence of breaths can be seen in this way, or you could use another image of your own. The emphasis is on the lightness of our breathing cycle, because when we are stressed, our breathing becomes heavy.

Activity 2:

Our next activity is about just *watching the air move*, as we breathe. It's one that I use often during stressful moments in the ED.

No interruptions.
Sit comfortably.
Eyes open or closed.
Don't worry about your thoughts – let them ramble.
We are just observing.
If you forget, try to get back on track.
No stress if you get distracted.
Just try and reach the two minutes.
And if you can, do this again.

5

CHECKLISTS

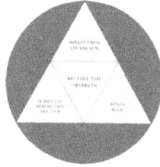

Motorcycles are not supposed to hit concrete barriers. The 17-year-old girl had been riding with her 19-year-old boyfriend, and they had struck slippery gravel on a corner in the road. Both had major injuries, and two teams of doctors and nurses were providing simultaneous assessment and resuscitation for the two riders. I was leading the team looking after the 17-year-old girl.

Roles had been clearly allocated. Team Leader, Airway, Breathing, Circulation, Procedures, Scribing... each role with specific assessment and action roles, and each role reporting regularly back to the Team Leader, whose job was to synthesise everything, plan the next steps, and ensure that nothing is forgotten.

With her multiple injuries, we had several things to do at once. The rapid IV replacement of her blood loss was a priority, even while we were still assessing the degree of injury.

Cognitively it was a very busy space. With so much going on there was opportunity for errors to creep in if we were not systematic and structured in our thinking.

Teams that handle multiple trauma all the time will reinforce these skills by frequent repetition. The hospitals that don't see trauma regularly need to develop and maintain such skills as best they can through other means, such as skills workshops or team simulations.

I was aware that the whole situation was very charged emotionally for me, and for the other nurses and doctors. The two motorcycle riders were so young, and yet so injured.

More than ever, we needed that calm thinking space, and to go through our checklists as we searched for injuries. Emergency training uses printed checklists, because we cannot physically remember all of these steps under the pressure of a resuscitation.

The resuscitation progressed; we restored her blood pressure, and it was safe to take her across the corridor to Radiology for a CT scan, or in a trauma environment, a "pan-scan" where the CT imaging starts at the brain level and goes right down through the neck, spine, chest and abdomen to the pelvis, sometimes even further to include the long bones of fractured limbs.

The conversations started with Orthopaedics, with General Surgery, and with the Retrieval Service who would take her by helicopter to a major trauma hospital 120km away, for the next stages of her care...

This is yet another reason for the *unshakeable mindfulness*. We must remember to be sequential, checking airway first, then breathing... all the way down to the feet and hands, looking for further fractures or skin injuries. As I worked my way through this young woman's diagnosis and treatment, I needed free bandwidth, uncluttered thinking space.

And that started by remembering the checklists for mindfulness, the breathing, the key words that brought me into calm.

Transitions back to those mindful spaces starts with **breathing,** which is one of our strongest techniques of transition, and **remembering,** a sacred recollection of our own previous, profoundly mindful moments.

All of this stuff is like a *remembering,* and the four areas in the diagram work towards that. We make that remembering process *unshakeable,* as if our lives depend on it, when we decide not to take any nonsense from our own unhelpful old thinking patterns. We clear the decks. Again. And again. And eventually we start to "get it" simply because we *keep on doing it.*

The Mindfulness Triangle

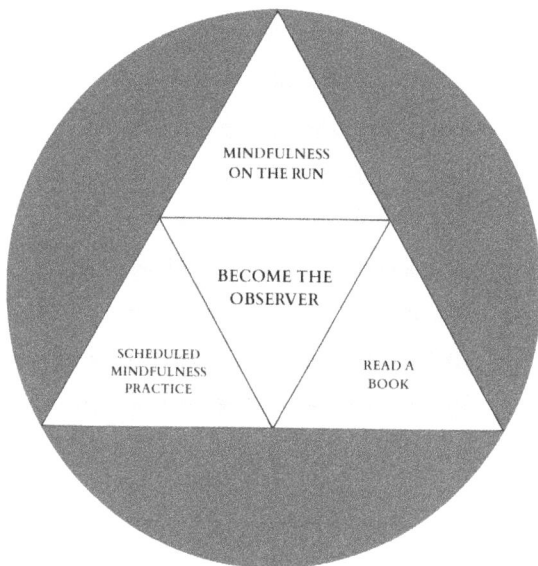

MINDFULNESS
ON THE RUN

BECOME THE
OBSERVER

SCHEDULED
MINDFULNESS
PRACTICE

READ A
BOOK

To highlight the diagram analogy:

1. We **OBSERVE** where we are starting from – the central triangle is crucial, as a start point.
2. We use a uniquely developed list of fast options for reaching a mindful state – **MINDFULNESS ON THE RUN** strategies, a checklist of alternatives including breathing and key mantras.
3. We have a background practice each day – **SCHEDULED MINDFULNESS PRACTICE,** which strengthens our mindfulness muscles; and
4. We access resources that inspire us and help us keep remembering that transitions to mindfulness are not only possible, but increasingly easy, as we just keep on doing the work - the **'READ A BOOK'** triangle.

Riding Bicycles and Turning Ships Around

- Schedule ten minutes of mindfulness meditation, once or twice a day.
- Be on the lookout for moments through the day when you can do a mindfulness on the run exercise.
- Constantly watch your thinking and replace old thoughts and emotional reactions in real time.
- Study the resources that inspire you every day, if possible.

Or to keep it even shorter, for emergency doctors like me with short attention spans...

- Schedule mindfulness practice sessions.
- Do mindfulness on the run.
- Watch thinking patterns constantly.
- Read a book.

Let's reverse some "traditional" concepts of learning when we think about mindfulness and meditation. I used to believe that mindfulness was about having to learn more stuff - more words to learn, sun salutes, trying to get into cross-legged positions, and other ideas that were hard to relate to.

Emergency medicine can also be about struggle, trying to push back the clock of the diseases we see, fighting to save someone with serious illness or injury. Mindfulness is the opposite. There's an *absence* of struggle, a progressive lightening of our effort, and this allows us great progress.

We aren't talking about loading on *more* ideas or concepts. Rather, we are talking about *unloading*. It is about *less*.

In the overloaded workplace of the hospital ER, mindfulness *must* rule. Keeping flow and smooth interactions with clinical colleagues is like applying oil to the cogs of a complicated gearbox. Nothing else would work.

None of us get it right all the time. Me included. We revert to old patterns - like anger, attack, and defensiveness - especially in the early stages of getting on the mindfulness learning curve. But increasingly, I would catch myself earlier and say an internal *Really? You're still doing this?*

We will push back against mindful thinking frequently at first, and our deeply entrenched stressful and angry patterns will try to grab hold of our thinking. But just like a child learning to ride a bicycle, who falls often, we learn *just as they do,* that the frustration of falling yet again needs to be put aside, to enable the next attempt to work better. We need to keep getting back on the bike.

There's a saying: "It takes a while to turn the ship around," and it does. So be patient with yourself. Just like water on the rocks in the stream, it takes time to carve out a new shape. But it need not take a lot of time if we commit to it and embrace the new way of approaching every conversation, every situation, and every thought we have.

"So be patient with yourself."

Day by day, thought by thought, we will develop an increasing ability to remember the new way, and turn the compass needle around to start the turning of the ship. This meditation and mindfulness stuff is fun, and the unexpected feedback you (yes, you), will receive from other people, about how wonderful they found your interaction with them, will act as positive reinforcement that this really does work.

Do the Remembering
See yourself
from outside,
Who do you see?
Do you see your *glow*?

Now, remember yourself,
so totally valuable,
so crucial in this creaking world.
What you have,
and what you *are*,
Is vital...
So, do the turning of the ship,
just turn,
towards that force of calm and care
that only wants you
to remember.
And then,
stand laughing,
In the steam-breath winter sun.
You're back,
There's work to do.

Cassette Tapes and Mindfulness

The decision in any moment is about imagining ourselves in two contrasting ways; the mindfulness, or positive way, versus the old negative way. It's easy to imagine ourselves in a negative way, and this tumbles through to what kind of experiences we will have each day.

Probably about 90 percent of our thoughts about ourselves are negative. We can so easily be suckered into negatively judging our bodies, our relationships, our bank balance, or our job situations. Little wonder that most of us are so open to anxiety and worry. The dominant internal narrative in most people is, as you would expect, predominantly negative.

Do you remember cassette tapes? Blank cassettes could be recorded onto multiple times. The new recording would simply rearrange the magnetic particles on the tape, erasing the previous recording.

Mindfulness is similar. We have a "recording" on our internal tape that keeps looping negative self-opinions, regrets about our past, and fears about the future. We are developing an unshakeable commitment, through mindfulness, to recording *another* narrative over the top. A new narrative that acknowledges something profound and important in ourselves, *despite* any appearances to the contrary.

At first, even thinking about ourselves in this way feels strange. But if we are going to make a lasting change, sooner or later we all need to make that choice to overwrite the tape, erase the old recordings, and replace them with new perspectives that are more useful to us.

Learning Through Repetition

When teaching my medical students how to suture a wound, or to make a plaster for a fractured bone, the sequences of each task need to be broken into bite-size segments. The whole procedure needs to be explained, demonstrated, and then repeated. Mastering any skill in medicine involves practicing over and over.

We all learn by repetition.

Each student is different, and some of them have natural aptitude for picking up these hand skills. Others need a lot of practice and explaining before they "get it".

We try something, we see that it did not work, we learn how to correct our approach, and then we make progress. Mindfulness and meditation are no different.

The Four Strategies

To get serious about really changing old patterns to more mindful patterns, we utilise the diagram with the "four strategies" of mindfulness.

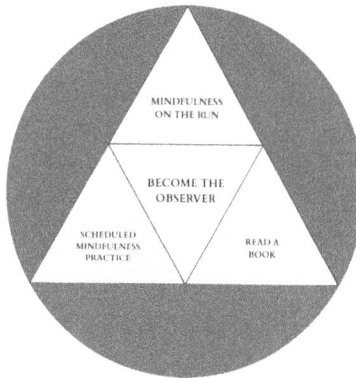

The Mindfulness Triangle summarises this whole book.

- Schedule some mindfulness practice.
- Find moments through the day for mindfulness on the run.
- Constantly watch thinking and replace unhelpful thoughts and emotional reactions in real time.

- Study a resource that inspires every day.

Strategies of Mindfulness

To remind us, mindfulness is about being observant of what is going on - in ourselves, in others, and around us. As an observer, we develop detachment, and we become less impacted by emotional reactions that wear us down.

Mindfulness strategies have a lot to contend with.

Our default way of thinking and reacting is, for most of us, a bit like a washing machine. Our thoughts are all over the place, and we seemingly have no control over feelings like irritability, anger, and fear.

To change all of this requires us to be *strategic*, and the initial mindfulness strategies are basically techniques to *distract* ourselves.

Scheduled Daily Mindfulness Practice

Or weekly, if it seems hard. But progress in any skill is related to frequency of practice. My medical students often hang around the ER, waiting for some action, and the ones that spend more time are rewarded with more practice opportunities, and their procedural skills reflect this.

Try each day, even if it is just for a few minutes, to help establish a discipline, and to train your mind into a very different pattern of thinking. Remember here that the "very different pattern of thinking" refers to perceiving your world with a forgiving and caring attitude to everyone, regardless of the apparent craziness on display. It also refers to the start of a new chapter in your emotional reactivity, where you will progressively *throw out* the default emotional reactions, like anger and fear, as you practice a mindful approach to *every* situation.

Waking up earlier allows you to develop the habit of setting up a positive and calm expectation for your day before you live through it. Be fully awake when you practice meditation or mindfulness exercises, so getting out of bed and sitting is preferable to snoozing off again as you meditate lying down.

And if you forget a day or three, it doesn't matter. Just come back the next day and keep at it. You will win through.

You can meditate with your eyes open, just looking at an object in an unfocussed kind of way, and not moving very much at all. Physical stillness makes for easier learning, especially at the start. There are beautiful movement meditations in yoga, tai chi, and other martial arts, such as the *kata* in karate. Reaching mindful spaces happens more easily when the movements are very slow and very smooth. And as you practice the same series of movements more and more, you will need less focus on "is it the left leg forward now?" thoughts, and as a result you will have more bandwidth to really sink down into the meditation.

Then there are the guided meditations, where you listen to a spoken voice, usually with music background. You are guided through a breath-slowing-down introduction, and perhaps a body-awareness sequence, which is a well-established mindfulness meditation approach. There are so many of these available, either in audio podcasts or YouTube and other social media, and most are free.

Experiment with these. We are all different. Everyone finds a style that works for them, and over time, you may swap around and explore different options. Try things. Be open-minded. Don't dismiss or prejudge different techniques, because there's an approach out there that is ideal for you.

In other words, we are all different, and the various available words and techniques that are a natural fit for one person, won't necessarily suit another. So, keep trying different stuff.

It's the same when I teach young doctors. If I see their eyes glazing over when I try to explain a concept in a way that is really obvious to me, I have to quickly change gears and come at it using another approach.

Eventually, it becomes unnecessary to have guided meditations, because we become our own guide, and silent meditation becomes easier and easier. We develop our own guidance system within. And *that* is a whole story in itself.

As you sit, you can listen to the guided meditation voice, or you can take the wheel yourself, and utilise one or several of the techniques we discussed in the earlier chapters, for reducing our inner mental and emotional *noise*.

Remember that image of pushing through the choppy waves near a beach until we get to the smooth water beyond...

Choose your mindfulness/meditation launch techniques from any or all of the suggestions below.

Scheduled Meditation... Some Tips and Tricks

- **Aim for a constant time of day and a regular place initially.**
- Try to avoid being interrupted.
- **Turn off phones.**
- Get comfortable and keep your body still for the practice session.
- **Shut your eyes or keep them open and still.**
- Start breathing in a timed pattern.
- **Let your breath rate slow down without effort or force.**
- Be aware of air movement through your nostrils, mouth, throat, and lungs.
- **Notice your body's weight and any pressure from contact with the chair or the floor.**
- Use a mantra or other word if you wish to accelerate a feeling of calm.
- **You can similarly use mental imagery that you associate with calmness.**
- Try stuff.
- **Visualise sinking down, through the ocean perhaps.**
- Use a guided meditation.
- **If you get distracted, remember that we all do, and simply return to the practice session.**
- Come out of each session slowly, using a return trigger like "coming up," for example, gradually opening your eyes, taking some deeper breaths, and slowly starting to move your limbs.

- Give thanks for the session if that feels like your style.
- Write down your reflections on the session if you wish.
- If you can, a short sleep after meditation is particularly restorative.

The last four ideas above reflect an important concept that when we are in meditation, it is ideal to *slowly* exit the practice session, rather than hurry things. It is also a lesson about taking the session seriously and being grateful for the gifts that each practice will bring us. Each time we practice, the benefits of meditation will be reinforced and expanded.

Unscheduled Mindfulness Practice: Mindfulness on the Run

We can be mindful at many moments through the average working day.

Other strategies that we can use at work or in the midst of our day include the slow walking exercise, a breath visualisation, and the observation of our emotional or physical state.

Constant observation of our reactions to triggers in the workplace or elsewhere such as catching ourselves mentally in that moment *before* we react, can avert unnecessary upset. To use the cassette analogy, whenever we catch ourselves starting to play the old thinking patterns, we can quickly "over-record" the tape with a mindful and forgiving perception of the person/situation/thoughts we are dealing with, and then respond completely differently.

Mindfulness on the run is about finding or creating short breaks in traffic to apply mindfulness techniques deliberately. It's a game we play with ourselves, to keep our thinking and reacting at our highest functioning level, as we go through the day. It's about staying present in a calm and deliberate way, all of the time.

Using walking slowly is a form of movement meditation, making our steps deliberately slow and smooth rather than the frenetic and jerky walking style we commonly see. Just making the effort to study the sensation of walking is a mindfulness technique all by itself. Feet on the ground, how the shoe feels, noticing balance shifting, being aware of the wind on your skin or the look of trees around you... it's a bit like waking up. Mindfulness is about deliberately noticing and observing, at both "inside us" and "outside us" levels.

Short mindfulness practices are great during the day to recalibrate our energy. Some hospital workplaces support this, acknowledging the staff health and patient safety benefits. Some even incorporate quiet rooms specifically for meditation periods, including an ER in the largest hospital in Reykjavik, Iceland.

Mindfulness on the run is about going through our day in a more *awake* state, quietly aware of everything around us.

Of course, if you are scheduling practice sessions on a regular basis, your mindfulness on the run moments will help you to remember the techniques you are experimenting with in the longer practices, and the whole "rebalancing as you pause" process becomes very efficient and time effective.

It's your move.

It's about making these strategies *unshakeable.*

Our daily lives provide the perfect training ground to help us
return to our own sense of peace.
We may not appreciate this at all, right now.
Nonetheless, we each have the same potential to react from a
place of calm, at all times, and in all situations

Watching Our Thoughts Constantly

Mindfulness for ten minutes a day, or once a week, or when
we go on a health retreat and meditate for a few days is a
start, but we can really accelerate the benefits if we start to
think in this way throughout *every* day and even through
every hour.

Our minds are amenable to new learning, new patterns, new
reactions.

We can certainly add to the difficulty by sending ourselves
thoughts like *It's impossible to change this. It's just the way I am,
and besides, my whole family is the same.* Or we can start a new
recording on the "cassette tape" that is our constant inner
loop of self-talk.

Take back the wheel, or alternatively just keep complaining
about someone else's driving. Whether we attribute our
default reactions to our upbringing, to our partner who
refuses to change their ways, or to life in general being
unkind to us, we *do* have the choice about how we run this.

And as I tell my medical students, true learning comes down
to *repetition* of the subject material.

- *Habits* are our natural individual tendencies in thinking or behaviour.
- We *can* change these, with dedication, if we perceive enough potential benefit to ourselves.
- *Repetition* of the new habit helps reinforce and stabilise our new thinking patterns and reactions.
- As they strengthen, they will become our *automatic* reactions.
- Each day gets easier, less reactive, and a lot more enjoyable.

It's probably clear by now that *regularly* looking at this "thinking stuff" is an essential element of changing our whole life over to a more mindful focus. It makes sense, because otherwise, it is equivalent to a language student who spends a few minutes in class practicing and does nothing at all in between those practice periods.

And it is through our own "thinking change" that we become more effective as agents of change.

6

NEXT LEVEL

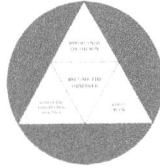

She presented to the ER describing feelings of depression and a serious intention to harm herself. Fresh razor lines and clotted blood are visible on each wrist, so I believed her. It was a busy Monday in ER, but she needed our care as soon as possible. 'Susan' (not her real name) was angry; angry at us for keeping her waiting, angry at us for not caring enough, and angry at her mental health care team for trying to provide her follow up by telephone rather than face-to-face. Angry that none of us could "fix her", she shouted at us.

Finding a spare room to talk with her was the first challenge. And then the triage nurse came over, selecting me and asking if I could see Susan. Part of me groans, knowing that I already had too many tasks underway, too many patients in that "half worked up" place where many decisions and investigation results are all happening at once...

But the other part says, "Yes, of course." I was the most appropriate doctor for this situation, because of my experience, but more so because of mindfulness. The other patients will just have to wait.

The conversation started with Susan. Perhaps not so much a conversation at first, but a type of attentive and non-reactive "listening", just sitting with her as her frustration tumbles out, washing over me.

The "old me" would have taken offence, reacted to the triggers, felt the muscles and body language changing into defensive mode.

But not now. Unshakeable mindfulness. Realising that my most effective operating space is from stillness. Susan could feel this quietness, even as her loud words came flooding out. She agreed to the proffered coffee and biscuits as her outpouring continued. I noted that her wrist wounds weren't bleeding. We would need to sort them out soon.

Mental health emergencies require the most senior nurses and doctors; the conversation has to go well, so in this one, our junior Hospital Medical Officer just "sits in" and observes, as I do most of the talking and listening. With some of these very complex consultations, we can't even have medical students or junior doctors in the room, because the patient will react anxiously to the very presence of someone else watching.

There are nurses and doctors who are comfortable in the 'mental health space', and others who are not.

I used to be in that latter group, but as a result of my exposure to a large number of ER patient consultations, I changed. I developed more compassion. But it was the mindfulness practice that brought it all together.

Poor outcomes result from poor quality interactions between clinicians and mental health patients. Poor outcomes can mean that someone leaves the hospital and commits suicide. The stakes are high, and the conversation matters so much. It really does matter, despite the pressure of my other patients who also needed me back there, collating their blood results, reading the CT result, ringing the consultant to arrange admission to the ward.

After a long conversation, Susan is calm. We cleaned and dressed her wrist wounds, arrange antibiotics and telephone the Psych team... then back to the other patients.

During the conversations like this, there's no road map. Yes, I know that there are some mental health lectures about how to verbally "de-escalate" an agitated patient, and how sometimes we need to use medication to sedate or reduce their anxiety levels.

But all of those structures are just the start; knowing which words to say, when to be silent and listen, and which questions will be appropriate – it's an intuitive situation and more of a *gut-feeling in the moment*. Because if we get it wrong, we can easily make false steps, and the link breaks. Once again, this bringing of *intuition* to the clinical moment is a quite deliberate skillset, one grown out of conscious mindfulness.

In an ER psych consult, there comes a point where we always contact the mental health team. The ongoing care and risk assessment is done by them because their training and skills are at a much higher level than ours. It may be a face-to-face consultation in the ER, or it may be a phone conversation now between the patient and the mental health clinician. Sometimes, it is an inpatient admission.

In each case, the accuracy of decision-making depends on the *quality of the communication* between ourselves as the ER care team, and the person who comes to us seeking mental health care at a time of crisis. We have to bring our "best game", and take enough time, despite the other patients whose needs temporarily must take second priority...

Of course, none of this happens by accident. Skills and intuition are present in all of us to varying degrees, because of our family backgrounds and life experiences. But we can deliberately develop them further. These are crucial in the ER environment, or in any conversation really, but particularly with someone in a mental health emergency.

Mindful Leadership

So, as we come into the final chapter, let's get clear about why this all matters, and how conscious mindfulness can take us to "next level".

Let's look at what makes a *great leader*. Because unshakeable mindfulness is closely related to the qualities of leadership. Look at the great leaders through history, and you'll see mindfulness in action.

The qualities of a good leader are many, but let's look at *three key qualities.*

1. **Skills**
2. **Stillness**
3. **Care**

But first let's compare ego-driven leadership with mindfulness-driven leadership.

All leaders need **skills**, and in the ER it's a combination of *technical* skills – clinical knowledge, examination skills, clinical reasoning, interpretation of investigation results, and correct treatment decisions – and the *non-technical* skills, which are of course our focus in this book.

The **stillness** of a great medical leader is the *radiance* that settles a resuscitation team, that invites high levels of *reciprocal trust,* and that *reduces* stress and psychological trauma from high-pressure clinical environments.

And the third word, **care**, is the bedrock of great leadership. A "non-targeted" care, for every person that the leader is dealing with – patients, colleagues, and families. We look after each person in the room. We could also describe this as *emotionally intelligent* leadership.

Developing leaders show these values or qualities to some degree but are not as conscious of this. This is the group who need development in any organisation, and the ER is no different. Talent needs to be nurtured and held onto.

Leaders have a choice, about whether to grow and consciously develop their skills. To stay current with the technical skills in emergency medicine, we need to maintain habits of life-long study and skills training. Meditation and mindfulness are no different.

Great leaders also have self-awareness: they see how important their own inner guidance is, and they demonstrate the above qualities in the way that they talk to others and make decisions. They inspire us, and they understand that each day, and each conversation, will provide further opportunities to contribute to the well-being of others. They consciously and deliberately practice the *"unshakeable mindfulness"* on which this whole book is based.

In my tutorials, I tell the junior medical staff and medical students to look at themselves as "clinical leaders in training". To look at the qualities of their own role-models, and to develop the same qualities that inspire them.

And you've probably figured that we are *all* leaders, that we all need to think of ourselves as leaders, growing into our full potential.

So, it's the last chapter, and here are some key "take home" ideas...

1. Use the mindfulness triangle – minute-to-minute mindfulness, daily scheduled practice, self-awareness at all times, and searching out inspiration sources.
2. Get a total handle on your emotional reactivity – control your response to triggers and anything else that irritates you.

Don't React to Triggers

A lot of people operate in an unconscious way throughout their entire lives. Stimulus. Reaction. Stimulus. Reaction.

Stress and oscillating emotional reactivity have negative effects on us, as well as the quality of our relationships to others, and aspects of our bodily health also.

Sooner or later, sometimes *much* later, we tire of this, because the constancy of attack / self-defence reactions depletes our energy. Angry people never look "young for their age".

The next step of understanding is that we realise that we have a choice. At that split second between a stimulus and the following reaction, we have the option to decide how we will react and how we will think about the situation.

Unshakeable mindfulness puts us back in control, a bit like grabbing the tiller in a sailing boat. We agree to steer our lives again, to take agency.

If we practice mindfulness at the start of each day, we have *already* decided ahead of time what our reactions will be to every potential trigger, as the day unfolds. We can reinforce this at night, with meditation practice before sleeping.

We create the probability of our emotional experiences ahead of time.

With repetition, this becomes our new default mode of reacting to *any* situation. Other people will notice. You will get comments like "I can't imagine you ever getting angry." The benefits are so many, the most immediate being that in that triggering situation, you're perhaps the only person in the room who *isn't* being triggered. Your effectiveness at reaching a creative solution expands. Your influence on others grows.

Our reactions to *triggers* will increasingly come from a place of calmness and great care for our fellow humans. In other words, much less anger, much less time spent in irritability.

We will all walk this road.

Steer the Boat

Our pathway towards a sense of peace is instinctive, even if we don't consciously understand why. As one example of *unconscious mindfulness*, we may not think of surf fishing as a spiritual journey, but we certainly are aware that we "feel better" when we are standing on a windy beach, watching the tip of the surf rod for any movements. Our mind spins down, and this is a beginning form of mindfulness.

But having said that, once we consciously decide to really go for this path, things really accelerate. The *unconscious mindfulness* is a bit like that sailing boat without anyone at the rudder. Occasionally, it will go in the right direction.

Conscious mindfulness, is when we put together the observation of our own lives, minute by minute, and we add the mindfulness-on-the-run strategies and also the daily scheduled practice sessions. The boat is finally steering straight.

And when we decide, as eventually we all will, to make this our compass for the rest of our life, it becomes *unshakeable*.

The Mindfulness Triangle

It's time to revisit the Mindfulness Triangle in more detail. It's not the *only* way to conceptualise mindfulness, but it certainly works for me as a busy ER Physician and Medical Educator. It's also applicable outside the hospital in "normal life".

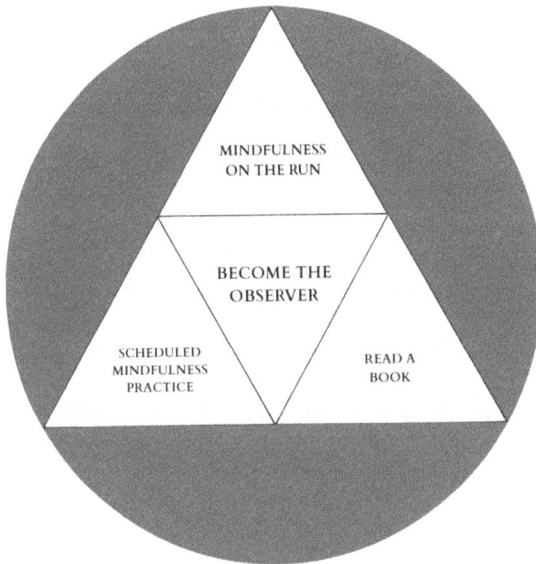

Put In The Work

The four elements involve us putting in the work. The curious discovery we each will make, is that any effort put in *within any* of the four triangles shown above has a magnifying effect in the *other* triangles as well.

In other words, a program of early morning scheduled mindfulness influences our thinking beyond this time, as we go through the day. Automatically, we will start to remember the strategies of "mindfulness on the run", and bring our mindful reactions to triggers, as it were.

The patterns become automatic and require less and less active thought on our part. Sometimes, we will get angry or annoyed. But the automatic observation of our thoughts kicks in, and we generate a "Really?" response. The anger is nipped in the bud, and we generate a more mindful response instead. Practice, practice.

Another example of this intermingling is how we will just *seem* to find resources (books, videos, meetings with strangers, conversations, etc.) that happen to have a gem or idea of some sort that is *exactly* what we need. It is almost as if we know just what we need, like a plant that absorbs the exact nutrients it needs for growth.

Behind it all, the *observation* of our thoughts becomes an automatic discipline that we will operate in most of the time. The meetings with people that we will have through our day are like mirrors; if the conversation goes well and we feel energised, we are probably responding and thinking in a mindful way.

If a conversation or thought leaves us feeling wound up or stressed, we have some work to do. Work on our own responses. It's all about the way we look at things. If we can achieve the internal reframing of what we think or see outside us, we move incrementally toward a state where we relate calmly to the world around us pretty much all of the time. We will become more influential and effective.

Also, the change in how we reframe the world we see is a change that we exert *in ourselves*. We are *not* demanding that others change their behaviour in order that we feel less stressed. Rather, we change the way that we think and react. We train ourselves, through repetition, to see the big picture or "top down" view of that other person or of the difficult conversation that we just had. It's a more compassionate view.

Maintain Momentum

When medical students learn CPR, we use the COACHED algorithm to minimise breaks in CPR and optimise the cardiac output achieved during chest compressions.

Similarly, if we have long breaks in between mindfulness practice, our progress slows, and we almost have to start again when we remember to resume our practice.

We all forget, and as we realise we have forgotten, then comes the remembering.

I was initially a very good *forgetter,* but also a good *rememberer* regarding my own mindfulness and meditation practice.

So, when we remember, we can get to work on *any* of the mindfulness triangles shown. Wherever we start, the progress builds, and it spreads to the other areas.

What *really* helps us remember faster is the fact that we *just feel better* when we are progressively living more and more of each day in a mindful way - scheduling practice, doing mindfulness on the run, observing our thoughts minute by minute, and allowing ourselves to pick up a book of learning that randomly catches our attention in the bookshop.

More importantly, we become better and safer clinicians, more measured and accurate in our diagnosis, and the "carriers" of a positive culture within our clinical teams.

And Above All...the Mindfulness Triangle is just not enough.

The mindfulness strategies and techniques are useful but, in a way, they are like the strategies and techniques of a horse trainer, who takes a wild and boisterous horse and gradually teaches it how to behave. Once the horse has become obedient, the next question is "So what do we do next?"

Purpose

One of the consequences of even the most superficial exploration of mindfulness is that these bigger questions about our *purpose* start to resurface.

One way of approaching this question is to describe two possible world views: the *material* worldview and the alternative *spiritual* worldview.

We need a model, because from the model, we make decisions which help guide our lives. We all have some kind of model about how life works and the things that are important to us.

Within a material worldview, mindfulness is perhaps explored for a specific purpose, such as being a way of helping with anxiety or sleep. Meditation techniques help with this. There's nothing wrong with a material worldview as such; it is a common starting point and a stage that we all must pass through, but it does not represent either our destination or our *purpose* here in the world.

Spiritual Worldview

Initially, our reason for coming to mindfulness may be to help with calming our brain and learning to overwrite old default emotional reactions. However, with repetition of the strategies of mindfulness, a journey starts automatically to take place within our mind that is unfamiliar, yet strangely familiar also.

It's like a journey to understanding ourselves in a whole new light. Let's call this view the *spiritual worldview,* but remember, it's not the title that matters.

It is a worldview that regards the care for other people as central.

Let's extend the Mindfulness Triangle to include the Circle of Care:

1. Mindfulness on the Run
2. Become the Observer
3. Read a Book
4. Schedule Mindfulness Sessions
5. The Circle of Care

The *Circle of Care*

The Circle of Care is the take-home message. With mindfulness strategies alone, we can go some way.

What is this *Circle of Care* anyway? Basically, it recognises that we use the strategies of mindfulness discussed previously, throughout each day.

In addition to this, the outer circle acts to remind us that we have a constant responsibility to the people we will meet each day, to respond to them in a mindful way, to ask our intuition for the best way to help them, and to fulfil our role in the best way we can.

The Circle of Care

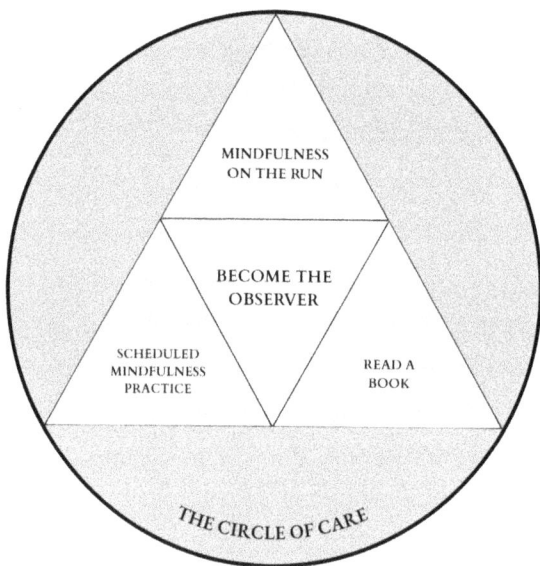

MINDFULNESS ON THE RUN

BECOME THE OBSERVER

SCHEDULED MINDFULNESS PRACTICE

READ A BOOK

THE CIRCLE OF CARE

The two parts are both essential and interlocking—the inner work and the outer work—we come to understand that we need the "mess and stress" to help us develop into our true potential.

Conventional mindfulness teaching is all about the Mindfulness Triangle. Spirituality is about the *Circle of Care*, as well, and you might use different language to describe the elements of the Mindfulness Triangle.

There are so many languages in our belief systems that describe the same phenomenon. And remember that we do *not* need spiritual beliefs of any sort for mindfulness to succeed.

The mindfulness concepts within the *Circle of Care* will certainly help us to reach our calm centre and to stay in it as much as possible. Of course, we will falter and forget these concepts, but that will slowly happen less and less. If we are mainly operating from mindful mode, our responses to others will be less reactive, less defensive, and less attacking. We become more compassionate and certainly useful.

Your Mission, if You Choose to Accept it...

We each have a role here. It will be different for you and for me. Each of us has a different skill set and unique abilities, which will equip us to solve different sorts of problems and to help different sorts of people.

As we remember to work more and more within the *Circle of Care*, supported by the strategies in the Mindfulness Triangle, we develop power and become very useful in this creaking world of ours.

And as we get a clear sense of what our internal compass needle is pointing to, we will then launch, with fledgling confidence, on our own journeys of *conscious mindfulness.* By becoming determined to hold this course, it becomes **unshakeable mindfulness.**

Another extension idea for this chapter is that *we are all destined to become teachers of these concepts.* Just as we are all destined to become leaders with the attributes of **skills, stillness** and **care.**

For as we truly learn anything, the next step is to *teach it* to those who we will meet and need our help, either consciously or by example in our day to day lives. I now know this to be true, and you will too.

Back to the ER...

Each day, in the ER, these concepts lie *behind* the way that I try to practice my profession. I am deliberately aware of the Mindfulness Triangle, the *Circle of Care,* and my Mission, as much of the time as I can be.

But above and beyond all of that, my way of thinking about and relating to others has at its centre the concepts in this book, as my *inner navigation system.*

It really works. And it can work for you too. This is the unshakeable mindfulness. It's a very deliberate and conscious process, based on the Mindfulness Triangle.

But beyond conscious mindfulness, we can all travel into developing our skills in *conscious care,* which is the *Circle of Care.*

We will be looked after if we focus on how best we can help others.

We Aren't Separate

No, we are all in this together. As tempting as it is to see our own journey and growth as our own private affair, we are linked. The idea that we can disregard the mass of humanity out there and just do our own thing makes no sense to me.

We affect each other by the way we *think* about others.

We most certainly influence and affect others by the way we *talk* to them.

It feels strange to think that we have such potential to change the world around us, but this is within our power, and it is our responsibility as humans on this planet.

Mindfulness is one very useful tool that we can use to strengthen this ability.

It's Not About You!

There's a commonly heard refrain in arguments: "It's not about you!" It's true; our life is *not* about us. It's about the *others*. *We* will be looked after if we focus on how best we can help the others who we encounter on our journey.

But the opposite is also true. Life *is* about us. Because this *Circle of Care* approach is actually *our* own best way forward.

So, in the end, *both* statements are true. The final idea. And it's a good place to bring this book to its end, with a closing poem and blessing.

And So We Close

You matter—
Much more than you
May even be aware of.
You are so important.
You are what I will name
A "crucial blessing"
To this world of ours.
And if your journey home
Is helped at all,
By ideas
That we've together touched,
My work is done;
I'll let these pages go.

MY DAILY PRACTICE

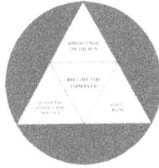

0600hrs
Make the Decision to Get UP!
In two hours from now I will walk through the ER automatic doors past the STAFF ONLY sign. And I could try to doze on further for another 30 minutes. But not now. There's a better way to launch the morning. Out of sleep. Drag the brain awake.

Sitting up vertically on the bed, the better position for morning meditation.

Watch any distracting thoughts, over-ride them, start the body scan anyway, and build a breathing meditation. It takes a few minutes to slow the thinking pattern down.

0610hrs
Meditation Time
This is my scheduled meditation from today at 0610, on a cold winter's morning: eyes shut, sitting on the bed.

First breath
Hold it
Explore the stillness between
This breath
And the next breath.
There's a familiar peace.
It's just like
Tuning the radio,
Locking on
To the frequency I seek.
The frequency of calm.
Setting this frequency.
This will be my default for
The whole day.
Every conversation will be held
From this frequency of calm.
And in it,
I will ask
What are the words to use?
How can I
Best help this person in front of me?
A few more breaths,
Enjoying the meditation space
Setting up another day
Then easing back to 'waking world'
Allow the normal thoughts in.
Stretch limbs and start to slowly move.

Soon it will be shower time and the day commences.

During meditation, an image came today...it was an idea of every cell in my body being like a tiny compass. With each in-breath, all of those compass needles rotate to point south, and with each out-breath, the needles all flip to point north. It's a fun visual image as I cycle through the breaths, going from <u>normal thought</u> through <u>early stages</u> to <u>deep calm</u>.

These little 'clues' can just arrive out of 'nowhere' to help us on our way. I think it works for anyone, if we start to watch for them. They're not really random, but that's a discussion for another day.

0640hrs
Letting Go of What Drains Good Energy

The "Be the Observer" opportunities come continuously; in case you're asking. In every thought actually. As I get ready for work, I am thinking about a work colleague that I was irritated with yesterday. It's time to 'clean up' those thoughts, to forgive the person and see them in a kinder light. It helps me if I can do that. The old 'what you give, you will receive' adage. It's the 'continually polish the lens' idea. 'Be the lighthouse'. It's simple enough affirmation stuff, but I find this really hard sometimes. Less so now, because of repetition.

0720hrs
Read (or listen) to a Book

Driving, I listen to the podcast on A Course in Miracles. The theme today in the lesson is forgiveness. I can certainly use these ideas. This is the '<u>read a book</u>' part of the mindfulness triangle, finding our own sources of inspiration, and pausing a while to listen to or read something that inspires us and educates us about our own growth.

0740hrs
Setting up the Day for Success
Moving through the carpark, having driven to the hospital across town in a state of calm, it's time to build an image of how well the coming day will progress. Sure, it's going to be busy, with too many patients and not enough beds at times, but the interactions will go well. It takes the *passivity* out of our daily experiences if we think like this. You guessed it... 'mindfulness on the run'.

0755hrs
Mindfulness on the Run
Into the emergency department, the first of many conversations, many procedures, X-Rays to analyse and blood-test results to integrate into making diagnoses. Teaching students, mentoring the interns, editing their notes, questioning their clinical reasoning. Modelling kindness, in every meeting whether with a cleaner or a patient or a senior colleague. Same. <u>Mindfulness on the run</u>.

1230hrs
The Danger Zone
–Unshakeable Mindfulness is Critical
Towards the middle of most days, the place is in overload. We might be on 'by-pass' by now, diverting ambulances. I have more patients than I would want, as do the other doctors. This is the risk-management issue of simply having too much work and not enough resources. This part of the day will settle after a few more frenetic hours. Many larger EDs don't really leave this state – they are overloaded for the entire 24 hours of each day.

1430hrs

The re-calibrations through the day are brief moments or minutes when I can do a few mindful breaths, because my brain is conditioned through enough practice to instantly go to calm when I start the slow breaths. Other options include slowly walking over to X-Ray for a verbal report, being an observer of the pressure as each footstep lands and takes off. The sending out of gratitude to the radiologist, or the cleaner. It's second nature now. It is like oil on the wheels and creates the mindful workplace.

1945hrs

At the end of the shift, I am tired. A deliberate slow walk back to the car. Sitting in the car I get the first 'closed-eye time' in the last 12 hours. It's like oxygen. Sitting in the car, eyes closed, just letting a meditation *come and find me* for a practice session before I fire up the engine and head home. After 15 minutes or so, I slowly return to <u>normal thought</u> and am ready to go home, to start the evening of cooking and conversations with my partner.

2015hrs

The meditations configure themselves around me, as I practice each day. As if the meditation itself 'knows' in some strange way exactly what my brain needs to re-balance and relax. Meditation starts off with 'transition systems', like breathing patterns, mantras, yoga movement, music or reading a passage in a book. But it all washes away in the end. The reflexes of transitioning from <u>normal thought</u> to <u>deep calm</u> become so strong, that we hardly need any of these transition devices. These aids to transition are essentially ways to distract ourselves away from our frenetic <u>normal thought</u> system. What increasingly becomes a trigger for rapid transition is, firstly, holding our eyes closed, and secondly just becoming physically immobile for a few minutes. Our brain is amenable to training and repetition, just like any muscle.

2045hrs

Making steamed vegetables again for the two of us. Mediterranean diet. Lining up the knife, the peeler and the chopping board. It's very Zen. Those monks are onto something. The precision and peace of peeling, slicing, adding and steaming. Knowing that the whole process is an affirmation of our health and what we take into our bodies. Cleaning up and washing dishes later is the same. Making it sacred. <u>Mindfulness on the run</u>. For a couple of hours my mind has been 'calling' me to meditate. That sounds so weird, but it is a thing.

2300hrs

At last, we start to settle in our night routines. And then into a <u>scheduled meditation</u>. Sitting on the couch, cross-legged, lights low. Eyes shut. Into breathing, a quick body scan. Send release to the neck muscles that carry tension so easily during my days. And then let the meditation come. If I use a mantra with in-breaths and out-breaths, it might be a one-word mantra. Or part of a word. Feather-light use of any words, as that is what works to catapult me down to <u>deep calm</u>. Just soak in it. About half an hour. I think I even drifted into sleep at moments during that time. It feels amazing coming back to the room, relaxed, energised. Sleep will be quality sleep tonight.

0000hrs
Mixing sleep with meditation usually doesn't work for me. Because it becomes sleep. And I need the sleep. The meditation practice creates more effective restoration during sleep. So, I meditate before bed, rather than in bed.

0200hrs (or thereabouts...)
But occasionally weird stuff happens right in the middle of the night. I come awake and it feels like a moment to go straight into meditation, as if there's some kind of inspiration ready to 'come through'. And the feeling of being suspended in completely profound calm sweeps over me, and I don't even feel tired. After maybe 45 minutes (it was pretty late, so this is a guess), I come out of meditation and settle back to conventional sleep.

0300hrs (I think)
I don't understand all of this, not by any means. It's a learning curve, but I know that it all makes me more and more effective in my roles during each day, as a partner, as a father and grandfather, as a doctor and a teacher, an administrator, and a mentor.

0600hrs
Didn't we do this already?!

SUGGESTED READING

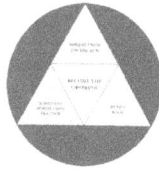

General Mindfulness:

Kabat-Zinn, J. (1990). *Full Catastrophe Living: Using the Wisdom of Your Body and Mind to Face Stress, Pain and Illness.* Delacorte Press.

Kabat-Zinn, J. *Wherever You Go, There You Are: Mindfulness Meditation in Everyday Life.* Hyperion.

Shapiro, S.L, & Carlson, L.E. (2009). *The Art and Science of Mindfulness: Integrating Mindfulness into Psychology and the Healing Professions.* APA.

Williams, M.,& Penman, D. (2011). *Mindfulness: An Eight-Week Plan for Finding Peace in a Frantic World.* Rodale.

Mindfulness Authors:

Deepak Chopra
Dr Wayne W Dyer
Gary Zukav

Meditation and Mindfulness Apps:

(Apple and Android)
Treat App: (free app)
Happier App: (paid app)
Headspace App: (paid app)
Calm App: (paid app)

Other Books:

A Course In Miracles. (2012). Sparkly Edition. Borderland Foundation.
Bach, R. (1970). *Jonathan Livingston Seagull*. Macmillan.
Dean, A. (2017). *Moving Light - Meditation Journeys*. Balboa.

CONNECT WITH DR ANDREW DEAN

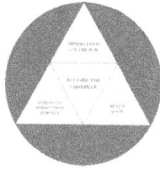

If you would like to hear from me personally please go to meditationformedics.com and sign up. I look forward to you joining us.

Dr Andrew Dean official website:

ACKNOWLEDGMENTS

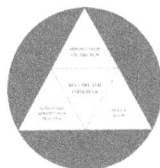

This book would not be here at all without the support, love and tolerance of the many individuals who have inspired and helped me along the way.

Firstly, to my partner Diane - my soulmate and teacher who encourages me each day to grow in every way. Thank you. To our beautiful children Lauren, Sally and Julian - thank you. Additional thanks to Lauren, for your graphic design skills. To Sally and her partner Phil, thank you also for your incredible photographic skills, as seen on my website.

To my publisher, Michelle Simone and the team from Hill of Content Publishing, a sincere thank you. You had faith in this book, and your many editorial suggestions have progressively sculpted the final book we see today.

To the remarkable individuals already practising mindfulness in my clinical workplace, you know who you are. Your level of conscious care for your patients and colleagues contributes so much. Thank you.

And to you, the reader, thank you. This book was primarily written that it be read by individuals who were seeking change in their own lives. I hope that this book fulfils that function.

www.ingramcontent.com/pod-product-compliance
Lightning Source LLC
Chambersburg PA
CBHW040756220326
41597CB00029BB/4936